IMMUNOLOGICAL
TECHNIQUES USING
FISH MODEL

A Laboratory Manual

A Manual for a Laboratory Course on Immunology
(in Life Science Programmes at Bachelors and Masters Levels on Biotechnology,
Microbiology, Biochemistry, Biology, Zoology and related subjects in Life Sciences)

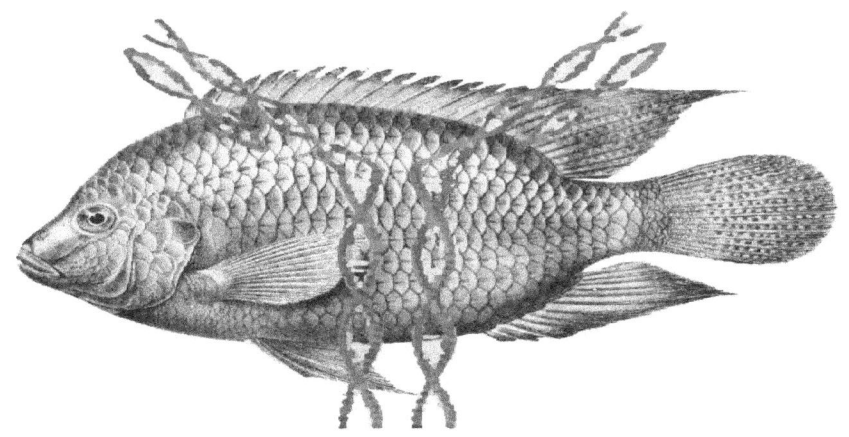

IMMUNOLOGICAL
TECHNIQUES USING
FISH MODEL

A Laboratory Manual

Prof. Dr. R. Dinakaran Michael, Ph.D.

Dean of Life Sciences and
Director, Centre for Fish Immunology
Vels Institute of Science, Technology and Advanced Studies,
Pallavaram, Chennai – 600117, India

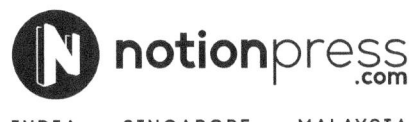

INDIA • SINGAPORE • MALAYSIA

Notion Press

Old No. 38, New No. 6
McNichols Road, Chetpet
Chennai - 600 031

First Published by Notion Press 2018
Copyright © R. Dinakaran Michael 2018
All Rights Reserved.

ISBN 978-1-64429-633-2

Dedication

This manual is dedicated to my wife Kamali, daughter Leena and son Rajeev who have been providing me, all these years, with an excellent and loving milieu by His Amazing Grace which also has sustained and guided me throughout my life.

FOREWORD

This manual on "Immunological Techniques using Fish model-A Laboratory Manual" is the outcome of long years of experience in teaching Immunology to Masters Students in The American College, Madurai by Professor. R. Dinakaran Michael, Dean of Life Sciences, Vels Institute of Science, Technology and Advanced Studies (Deemed to be University), Chennai. The various experiments detailed in this manual have also been used by Prof. Michael to train participants from different parts of India in several national level workshops. Moreover, on the basis of his significant contributions to Fish Immunology, Dr.Michael has been recognized internationally (A short history of research on Immunity to infectious diseases in Fish, Development and Comparative Immunology, 2013).

Ever since the discovery of the function of the thymus by Dr. JAFP Miller and the formulation of the clonal selection theory by Sir Frank Macfarlane Burnet during 1960s, the field of Immunology witnessed a phenomenal growth, thus recognized as an independent discipline in Biomedical Sciences. Further, Immunology has been taught as an essential part of teaching programmes for students of Biological and Biomedical Sciences. The usual practice is to make use of mice, rats, and rabbits to demonstrate in the laboratory, the various concepts of Immunology. Since the approved animal house facility is not available in most of the teaching institutions in India, the desired laboratory classes could not be conducted. This manual by using a fish model satisfies the requirement of teaching laboratory classes.

Prof. Michael has ably attempted to cover several aspects of laboratory course in Immunology which would complement the concepts taught in theory classes. This comprehensive manual includes a series of simple experiments on the organization of lymphoid organs, various types of immune responses, the methods to measure humoral and cell-mediated-immunity as well as vaccine development and non-specific immune responses using a fish model.

I consider it a special privilege to have had an opportunity to write this foreword in appreciation of the remarkable contribution in preparing this manual by Prof. Dinakaran Michael.

Prof. VR. Muthukkaruppan

Formerly, Professor of Immunology, Madurai Kamaraj University, Madurai
Former Vice Chancellor, Bharathidasan University, Trichy
Advisor-Research, Aravind Medical Research Foundation, Madurai

ACKNOWLEDGEMENTS

I wish to record my sincere gratitude for the support, encouragement and guidance I received from my teacher and mentor, Prof. Dr. VR. Muthukkaruppan FNA, FASc, Advisor-Research, Aravind Medical Research Foundation, Dr. Venkataswamy Eye Research Institute, Madurai-625020, India for conducting a National level Academies' Refresher course on 'Immunology Laboratory Techniques Using Fish Model' at Vels Institute of Science, Technology and Advanced Studies, Chennai in December, 2016, for suggesting very valuable modifications in the draft manual after diligently going through the entire manuscript and for writing an excellent foreword for the manual.

I am very thankful to our Chancellor, Dr. Ishari K Ganesh for inviting me to Vels Institute of Science, Technology and Advanced Studies, Pallavaram in 2010 to establish the Research Centre for Fish Immunology and provided me with a good working laboratory and an excellent fish keeping facility. This invitation gave me an opportunity to continue my fish immunology research for the last nearly eight years and to conduct Academies' two weeks Refresher Course on 'Immunology Laboratory Techniques Using Fish Model' in 2016 which resulted in this manual for the benefit of all the teachers and students of immunology in this country and elsewhere.

I am grateful to my mentor, Prof. Dr. T. J. Pandian, FNA, FASc, FNASc Former ICAR National Professor and INSA Senior Scientist, School of Biological Sciences Madurai Kamaraj University, Madurai-625021, India for his enthusiastic guidance and support for all my academic endeavours including some of my major research projects which sustained my research in fish immunology, all these years.

I am thankful to Prof. Dr. Nirmala Jeyaraj, Ph.D. Former Principal, Lady Doak College and presently, Secretary, Rev. Jacob Memorial Christian College Ambilikkai-624612, Dindigul Dt. for inviting me to Lady Doak College for establishing a research centre for Fish Immunology and providing me with excellent laboratory and fish keeping facilities and an environment conducive to doing quality research and conducting quite a few national level immunology workshops.

I am thankful to Prof. Dr. RM. Pitchappan, FASc, FAMS, Former Professor and Head, Department of Immunology, School of Biological Sciences Madurai Kamaraj University Madurai-625021 who is always appreciative of my scientific endeavours and efforts and also prompt in giving constructive suggestions to take them to higher levels. I earnestly appreciate the contributions of my former colleagues Mr. S. Suriakumar, Dr. Navaneetha Kannan, late Dr. Kumarasamy and my doctoral students, Mr. Isaac Arunkumar, Dr. M. Prabakaran, Lt. Cl. Dr. C. Binu Ramesh, Dr. L.D. Devasree, Dr. Catherine P. Alexander, Dr. M. Divya Gnaneswari, Dr. John Wesly Kirubakaran, Ms. Christy Babita, Dr. Priyatharsini Rajendran, Ms. S.Kalaivani Priyadarshini, Dr. B. Ramalakshmi, Ms. Omita Yengkhom, Mr. A.S. Parasuraman, Ms. K.S. Shalini for assisting in planning and conducting numerous national level training workshops on Immunological Techniques which ultimately resulted in developing this novel concept of using fish as a laboratory model to demonstrate immunological principles and also for assisting in various ways during the preparation of this manual.

I am happy to make a note of the good laboratory and technical assistance provided by Messrs M.A. Mazeedkhan, Ramesh Daniel, Parameswaran, Saravanan and Rameshkumar and Ms.Geetha for the successful conduct of the workshops referred above.

I am pleased to record my appreciation of the contribution by my grandson Chris Navin Samuel, a high school student who drew good pictures for some of the exercises in this manual using MS Paint.

Finally, I feel that I shouldn't miss this rare and relevant opportunity to record my gratitude to my teacher during my graduate studies, late Prof. J.C.B. Abraham, who inspired me by his excellent lectures to get me amply interested in biology and to my Principal, late Dr. M.A. Thangaraj who instilled in me some good values for life and work.

Prof. Dr. R. Dinakaran Michael, Ph.D.

Dean of Life Sciences and
Director, Centre for Fish Immunology
Vels Institute of Science, Technology and Advanced Studies
Pallavaram, Chennai-600117

WHY THIS MANUAL OF IMMUNOLOGICAL TECHNIQUES USING FISH MODEL?

The laboratory manual is novel and innovative in its approach and vast in its utility. The manual is very suitable for colleges and universities in India and other developing countries in the third world and of course, the rest of the world.

The manual is intended to be used for Immunology laboratory courses in

1. Life Science disciplines in Arts and Science Institutions (B.Sc. and M.Sc. in Zoology, Animal Science, Biotechnology, Microbiology, Biochemistry, and Bioinformatics etc.)

2. Life science disciplines in Engineering -Technology institutions (B. Tech and M. Tech in Biotechnology, Bioengineering, and Bioinformatics etc.)

3. Medical, Veterinary and Fisheries Institutions (M.B.B.S., BVSc., B.Pharm., M. Pharm., B.FSc, M.FSc etc.)

There is no frontier area in life science that has remained untouched by the subject, Immunology. Immunology plays rather a dominant role in modern biological, medical, veterinary, and fisheries sciences. The driving force for such a role is, the need to understand immunological basis of large number of infectious, autoimmune and malignant diseases; to develop effective prophylactic vaccines and immunomodulators for existing and newer infectious and other diseases of humans, cattle, poultry and fish; to practice immunotherapy involving cytokines like interleukins and interferons and antibody engineering products like chimeric/humanized monoclonal antibodies, plantibodies and immunotoxins and also to use immunological tests for diagnostics.

The subject of immunology has been introduced in undergraduate and postgraduate curricula of all the life science disciplines in science, engineering and technology institutions. Immunology is also a valued subject in medicine, veterinary science, and fisheries. The institutions offering immunology in their life science programmes have frequently expressed constraints in conducting immunology laboratory exercises due to lack of facilities like well maintained animal houses to keep the experimental animals like rabbits, guinea pigs, rats and mice and regular technical/ laboratory assistance to maintain these animals. All these issues are ultimately due to financial constraints. Further, there are constraints in terms of clearance from Institutional Animal Ethical Committee (IAEC) for using sufficient number animals like rabbits, guinea pigs, mice and rats for the Immunology laboratory exercises. The teachers of immunology also expressed the lack of an 'easy to use' immunology laboratory manual with simple techniques/procedures to demonstrate and explain the basic and important immunological concepts. These kinds of persistent constraints resulted in many institutions offering of an immunology course, even at post graduate level, without any worthy laboratory component.

With my fairly long experience in offering theory and laboratory courses on immunology for post-graduate Life Science students in this country and abroad and in doing research in fish immunology along with my experience of conducting many centrally sponsored national level training workshops on immunological techniques for young college/university faculty fellows and scientists, I thought it would be worthwhile to reach wider audience in this country and other countries by publishing the personally and time tested procedures, using a fish model (which is an excellent alternative to mammalian models to demonstrate the immunological concepts traditionally explained by using mammalian models) to overcome the above mentioned constraints in conducting immunology laboratory exercises.

Fishes phylogenetically were the first group of animals to have a lymphoid system with T and B cells and they were first to have 'invented' immunoglobulins, the so-called antibodies. They have been shown to have the immunological components, mechanisms and molecules found in higher vertebrates like mouse and man though in a simpler style. Hence, fish is an ideal vertebrate model for understanding and teaching the essential immunological concepts and perhaps other physiological concepts as well.

Using fish as a model to understand complex mechanisms underlying human systems is routinely practiced in many biomedical research areas. Over many years, biomedical scientists have developed zebra fish model for investigating many human diseases like cancer, cardiovascular diseases, retinal conditions and immunological disorders like acute inflammation and the same fish model is also used for developing potential and potent new drugs. The basis for such approaches is that disease phenomena can be better understood in whole (model) organisms rather than studying human cells in culture or molecules in test tubes. Hence, it is sensible and scientific to use fish as a model in an immunology laboratory course for understanding immunology of higher vertebrates including humans.

The fish species proposed to be used for the immunology laboratory course is tilapia (*Oreochromis mossambicus/niloticus*) which we have been using for a long time in our research and to teach theory and laboratory courses in immunology. The fish proposed is an inexpensive fish in India and a remarkably robust fish, readily adapting to available environment and food sources. It also tolerates wide range of water salinity (euryhaline) and temperature (eurythermal, 10 °C to38 °C). All these details mean that this fish can easily be maintained in a laboratory for experimentation. All one needs is a few 80 L plastic round tubs with water, a few simple aerators and feed pellets which can be easily prepared in the laboratory. The fish can be easily maintained by the students themselves.

This 'easy to follow' laboratory manual includes the procedures of many important immunological techniques. These techniques were repeatedly and routinely used in our department and research centre for fish immunology. We also used these techniques in many national level training workshops on immunological techniques we conducted and in particular, the recently conducted Two weeks Academies' Refresher Course on 'Immunology Techniques using Fish Model' in this university sponsored by the three major Science Academies of this country.

Most of these techniques, I strongly believe, can be introduced in colleges and universities in India and elsewhere in the world for laboratory exercises in immunology and perhaps in their teaching and research in immunology. We can offer our continued guidance and support for the users of this manual in their efforts in introducing these techniques in their teaching laboratories or for using these techniques in their research.

Prof. Dr. R. Dinakaran Michael, Ph.D.

Dean of Life Sciences and
Director, Centre for Fish Immunology
Vels Institute of Science, Technology and Advanced Studies (VISTAS)
Pallavaram, Chennai-600117.

CONTENTS

1. BASIC TECHNIQUES

This section includes some general and preparatory exercises like dissecting lymphoid organs in fish and separation of leucocytes from these organs, preparations of different kinds of antigens, Immunization of fish and fish bleeding technique.

1.1   FISH LYMPHOID ORGANS (THYMUS, SPLEEN AND HEAD KIDNEY)

Introduction

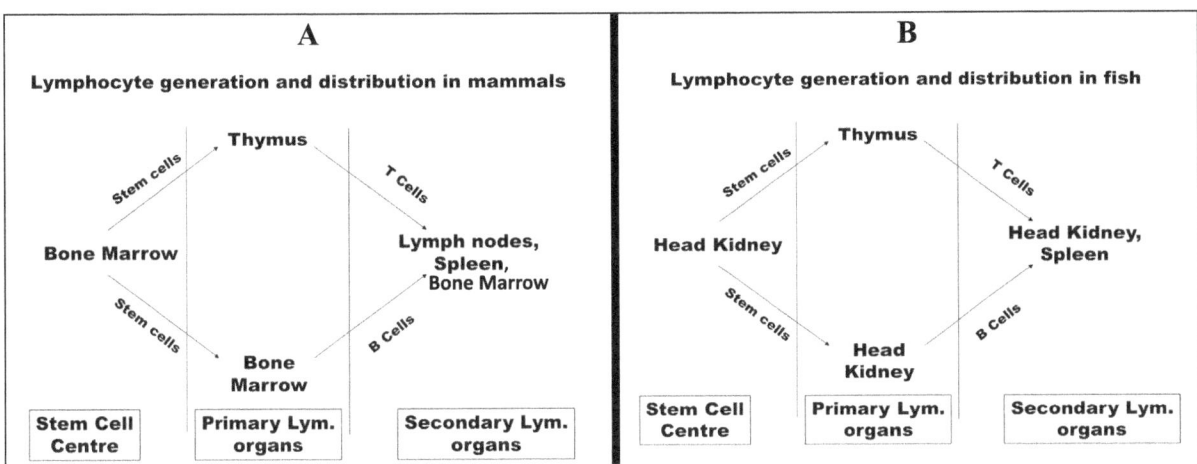

Figure 1.1   (A) Lymphocyte generation and distribution in mammals and (B) fishes

Lymphoid organs are unique to vertebrates. Lymphoid organs can be classified based on their function. In mammals, the 'central' or 'primary' lymphoid organs, Thymus, and Bone marrow are concerned with the production and processing of T-lymphocytes or B-lymphocytes respectively (in birds the B lymphocytes are generated from Bursa of Fabricius). Bone marrow is also the place of generation stem cells which are processed to become the T and B lymphocytes. The peripheral or secondary lymphoid organs, the spleen and lymph nodes (and also bone marrow) harbour the mature T and B cells and these organs play important role in specific immunity. Spleen acts as a filter for antigens that have entered blood circulation. On the other hand, lymph nodes act as a filter for antigens that enter through lymphatic circulation. In these organs, the earlyinteractions between the antigen and immune reactive cells (T and B cells and antigen presenting cells) occur.

Since, fish lack lymphatic circulation, lymph nodes are absent in them. Further they also lack bone marrow. In fish, the "head kidney" (pronephros) acts as the stem cell centre, primary lymphoid organ (to produce B lymphocytes) and also a secondary lymphoid organ. Thus head kidney functions as an equivalent of mammalian bone marrow. The head kidney and spleen are secondary lymphoid organs and they are rich in T cells and B cells. Hence, these organs facilitate the interaction of pathogens/

antigens with lymphocytes. Spleen and head kidney are ideal sources for macrophages, T-cells and B-cells. Generally, thymus is larger in young ones than in adults. In the present lab exercise, we will be observing the lymphoid organs in fish namely Thymus, Spleen and Head kidney.

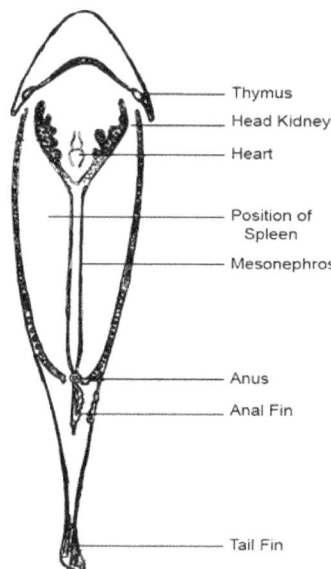

Figure 1.2   Relative location of three important lymphoid organs namely thymus, head kidney and spleen to that of other organs in Nile tilapia, Oreochromis niloticus. (Modified from Sailendri,1973)

Materials

- Dissection microscope
- Dissection tray and dissection board
- Large glass jar
- Table lamp
- Pins, Nails and hammer
- Scissors (large) and Scissors (fine)
- Small forceps (watch maker's)
- Pasteur pipettes

- Tilapia 30 g (As per requirement)
- PBS
- MS 222 (Tricaine mesylate/Tricaine methanesulfonate/TMS) or 2-Phenoxyethanol

Lymphoid Organs in Fish

All bony fishes possess a thymus and a spleen. In addition, the anterior or the head kidney also serves as stem cell centre, primary lymphoid organ and also as a secondary lymphoid organ.

Thymus

The thymus is a whitish opaque bilateral organ situated on both sides in the angle formed by the operculum and the dorso-lateral body musculature. It lies superficially in close association with the epithelial lining of branchial cavity. It measures 6 x 3 x 1 mm and contains $11\text{-}13 \times 10^6$ thymocytes in young tilapia of about 40g size. Macroscopically, this organ is elongated with its pointed end facing anteriorly and broader end posteriorly.

Procedure:

1. Tilapia of about 30 g is anaesthetized in 0.005% MS222 or 2-Phenoxyethanol (100 ppm)The gill cavity is washed with tap water to remove any debris.The fish is pinned onto the dissecting mat with the left side of the fish facing up.
2. Cut and Remove the operculum
3. The branchial epithelium is peeled off with the help of fine forceps to locate the thymus.
4. Thymus is seen as a whitish opaque organ in the angle formed by the operculum and the dorso-lateral body musculature, superficially in close association with the epithelial lining of that site of branchial cavity.

Note:

1. Thymus is seen clearly in young tilapia (20-40 g), not in larvae or old fish.
2. Thymus is usually seen at spring and summer better than during winter and autumn.
3. Due care is to be given to the fact that thymus is very small and easily damaged by hand or dissection tools during dissection.

A

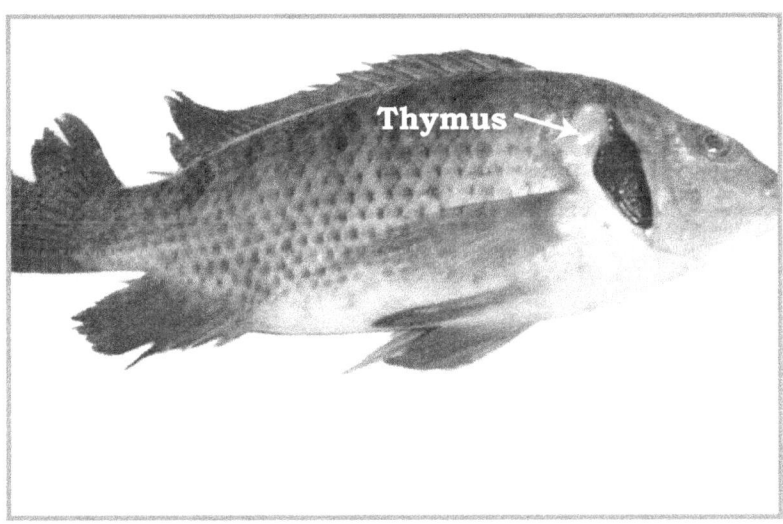

B

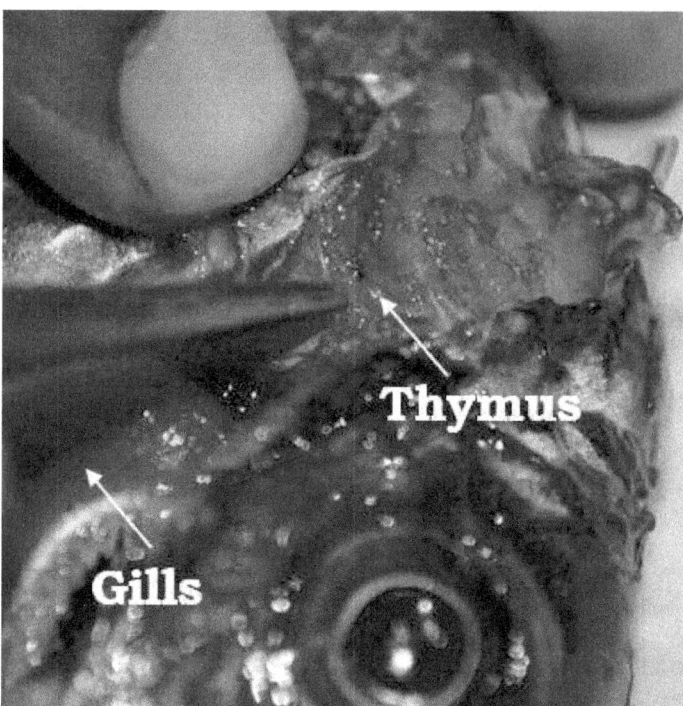

Figure 1.3 A. Lateral view of the *Oreochromis niloticus* fish showing the thymus (arrow) (Courtesy: Mona Nasr, Departments of Histology and Cytology, Banha University, Banha, Egypt). B. Thymus is shown as located on the superior edge of the gill cover/operculum (Courtesy: M.S.A Muthukumar Nadar, Karunya University, Coimbatore, India).

Spleen

The spleen is an elongated, flat structure, measuring up to 12mm in length and 1mm in thickness. It lies along the left side of the stomach, in close association with the pancreas. It is reddish brown in colour and contains of $5\text{-}9 \times 10^6$ white cells. Though spleen is also a secondary lymphoid centre, it is more erythropoietic than lymphoid in function.

Procedure

1. Anaesthetize 30 g size male fish in 0.005% MS222 or 2-Phenoxyethanol (100 ppm) and the rinse the fish in water to remove the anaesthetic. Lightly pat the fish dry on a paper towel.
2. Place the fish onto the dissecting mat. Cut the skin from the anal fin along the belly of the fish to the operculum.
3. Next, place the fish laterally and remove the gastrointestinal system from the body cavity of the fish.
4. The spleen is in the peritoneal fat, near the greater curvature of the stomach or the first flexure of the intestine. It is generally oval and flattened.

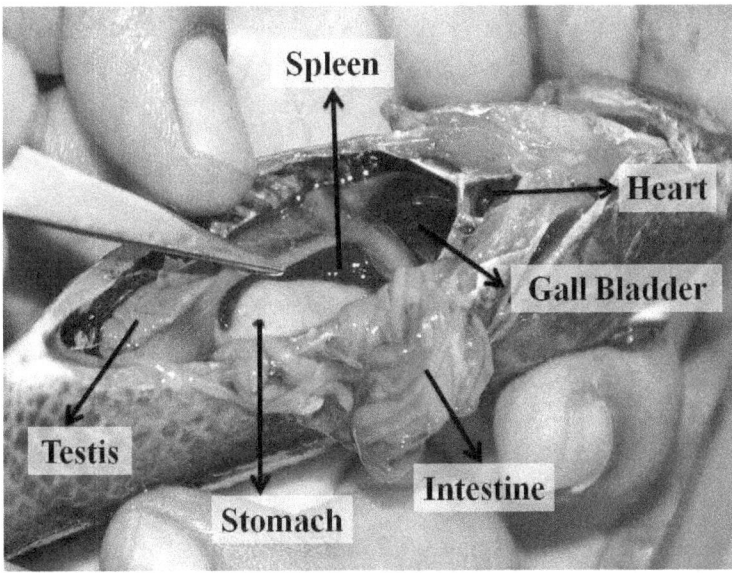

Figure 1.4   Ventral view of the *Oreochromis niloticus* fish showing the spleen. (Courtesy: M.S.A. Muthukumar Nadar, Karunya University, Coimbatore, India)

Head Kidney

It is the term given to the modified pronephros at the anterior end of the mesonephros, which lies in dorsal region of the body cavity, ventral to vertebral column, just outside the peritoneum. It extends from the level of thymus in the branchial region to the anterior end of the mesonephros. In adults, it measures about 8 to 15 mm in length. It is dark brown in colour and contains approximately $9 - 16 \times 10^6$ leucocytes. Head kidney of the fish not only acts as the stem cell centre but also as primary as well as secondary lymphoid organs.

Procedure

1. Anesthetize 30 g fish in 0.005% MS222 or 2-Phenoxyethanol (100 ppm) and the rinse the fish in water to remove the Tricaine. Lightly pat the fish dry on a paper towel.
2. Place the fish onto the dissecting mat. Cut the skin from the anal fin along the belly of the fish to the operculum.
3. Next, place the fish laterally and remove the gastrointestinal system from the body cavity of the fish.
4. Next, examine the swim bladder. The swim bladder consists of a posterior chamber, which is connected to the oesophagus via the pneumatic duct, and an anterior chamber, which is connected to the inner ear through the Weberian apparatus.
5. Remove and discard the swim bladder. Unpin the fish and re-pin it ventral side up to dissect the kidney, which is located along the dorsal body wall.
6. The kidney is a translucent pink structure associated with the dorsal aorta and pigmented cells. The kidney is divided into head, body, and tail regions (Figure 1.3).
7. Dissect out a piece of the kidney and place it in PBS. Tease apart the kidney tissue to reveal the renal tubules.

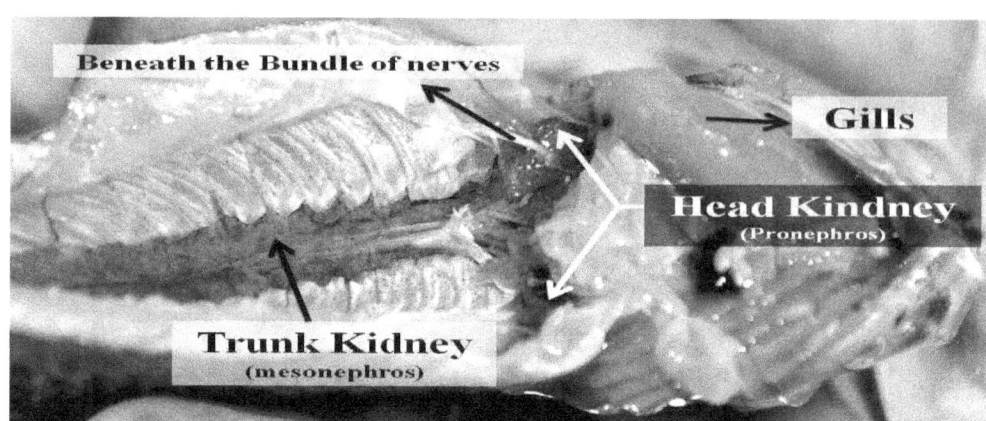

Figure 1.5   Ventral view of the *Oreochromis niloticus* showing the head kidney and trunk kidney along the dorsal body wall (Courtesy: M.S.A. Muthu Kumar Nadar, Karunya University, Coimbatore, India).

References

1.   Attia, H.F;* I.M.A El-Zoghby; *Mona N. A. Hussein and **H. H Bakry. Seasonal changes in the Thymus gland of *Tilapia nilotica*. 2010. Minufiya Vet. J. 7:1.

2.   Kumar G., Abd-Elfattah, A. and El-Matbouli. Identification of differentially expressed genes of brown trout (*Salmo trutta*) and rainbow trout (*Oncorhynchus mykiss*) in response to *Tetracapsuloides bryosalmonae* (Myxozoa). M. Parasitol Res. 2015. DOI 10.1007/s00436-014-4258-1.

3.   http://learninganimalphysiology.weebly.com/fish.html.

·· **Notes/Records** ··

.... **Notes/Records** ....

1.2 SEPARATION OF LEUCOCYTES FROM THYMUS, SPLEEN AND HEAD KIDNEY

Introduction

For doing various assays to test the effector functions of leucocytes such as Reactive Oxygen Species (ROS) or Reactive Nitrogen Intermediates (RNI) production by macrophages or Neutrophils, lymphocyte proliferation etc., the leucocytes from the lymphoid organs (such as thymus, spleen and head kidney) have to be separated and subjected to various procedural steps. This section describes the procedure for separating leucocytes from the lymphoid organs.

Materials

- Microplate reader (Biorad iMark)
- 96 well flat bottom plates
- 100 mm mesh nylon gauze
- 100 μm Nylon mesh
- Sterile centrifuge tubes
- Ice pack
- Neubauer chamber (Haemocytometer)
- Binocular microscope

- Tilapia 40-50g (As per requirements)
- Blood collecting medium (RPMI 1640 supplemented with 50 IU/ml Sodium heparin, 100 IU/ml Penicillin and 100 μg/ml Streptomycin).
- Wash medium (RPMI 1640 supplemented with 10 IU/ml Sodium heparin, 100 IU/ml Penicillin and 100 μg/ml Streptomycin).

Procedure

Separation of leucocytes from Thymus/Head Kidney/Spleen

1. The thymus/head kidney/spleen is dissected out aseptically and transferred onto a tube containing 2ml of blood collecting medium. The contents are mixed well and stored in an ice pack.
2. Using sterile forceps, the thymus/head kidney/spleen is placed onto the nylon mesh (100μm) mounted on a bottle.
3. With the help of sterile pestle (or glass piston of tuberculin syringe) the thymus/head kidney/spleen is gently mashed. Use excess wash media to wash of cells into the bottle.
4. The resulting single cell suspension is re-suspended with 2ml of wash medium in sterile tube and enumerated using Haemocytometer in a binocular microscope.

Note:

1. For performing viable cell count Trypan Blue (vital stain) exclusion can be used to avoid counting dead cells. Commercial Trypan Blue (0.4% in PBS, HiMedia) is

mixed with equal volume of cell suspension and counted in haemocytometer as soon as possible.

2. Live cells appear colourless and bright (refractive) under phase contrast microscope.

3. Dead cells stain blue and are non-refractive.

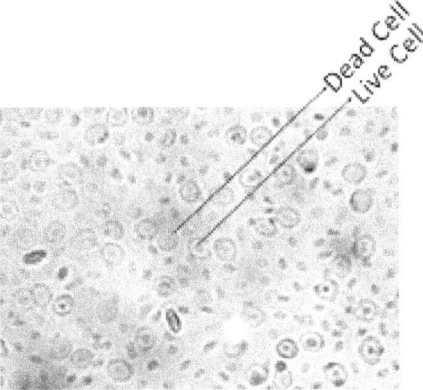

Figure 1.6 Trypan Blue exclusion test (Note the blue coloured dead cells and colourless live cells)

Reference

1. https://www.phe-culturecollections.org.uk/technical/ccp/cellcounting.aspx.

.... **Notes/Records** ....

1.3 PREPARATION OF ANTIGENS

Introduction

Nature and level of antibody response vary markedly according to the physical form of antigens. Generally, soluble antigens such as Bovine Serum Albumin (BSA) dissolved in saline are less immunogenic than particulate antigens like erythrocytes or even BSA aggregated by heat. Phagocytosis of antigen for processing and presentation is essential for an immune response. Susceptibility of particulate antigen to rapid phagocytosis is said to be the reason for more prompt and better response to particulate form of BSA (e.g. Heat aggregated BSA) than to its soluble form (BSA dissolved in saline). Administration of antigen incorporated (emulsified) in oil adjuvants (e.g., FIA – Freund's Incomplete Adjuvant – mineral oil) generally leads to enhanced response because of the slow release of antigen from oil droplets and the stimulatory effects of the bacterial components (if present in the adjuvant, e.g. FCA – Freund's Complete Adjuvant) on the immunocompetent cells.

A. Preparation of Erythrocyte Antigen – Sheep Red Blood Cells (SRBC)

Cellular antigens such as Sheep erythrocytes are complex antigens and they are usually, highly immunogenic in many vertebrates.

Materials

- Centrifuge (Remi table top)
- Haemocytometer
- 30ml glass syringe
- 18-gauge needle
- Conical flasks
- 15 ml graduated centrifuge tubes with conical bottom

- Alsever's solution (anticoagulant) (see Appendix)
- Physiological saline (0.15 M) (see Appendix)

Procedure

1. Sheep blood can be drawn from the jugular vein of sheep into sterile Alsever's solution using sterilized 30 ml syringe and 18-gauge needle. Sheep blood, as far as possible, can be collected aseptically into a conical flask containing Alsever's solution carefully during slaughtering of a sheep in slaughter house.

2. The Alsever's - diluted blood is immediately aliquoted in small conical flasks (50 or 100 ml) with additional Alsever's solution (final ratio, sheep blood: Alsever's 1:3 – 1:4). It is stored at 4°C in refrigerator.

3. Sheep red blood cells (SRBC) are prepared by washing sheep blood (stored in Alsever's solution) thrice in physiological saline by centrifugation at 3000 rpm for 10 minutes.

4. The pelleted/packed SRBC is resuspended in saline to the required concentration in terms of percent packed SRBC volume in the suspension.

5. The concentration of antigen can be checked by counting the SRBC in haemocytometer (The number of red blood cells in 0.1 ml of 25% SRBC is about 6 x 10^8 cells).

Note: To raise hyperimmune serum, fish must be injected with a priming dose of 0.1ml of 5% SRBC followed after 3 days by a booster dose of 0.1ml of 25% SRBC. This should be further followed after 2 or 3 weeks by another booster dose of 0.1 ml of 25% SRBC

B. Preparation of Bacterial Antigen – *Aeromonas hydrophila*

Live bacterial cells are usually inactivated by heat or formalin when used as antigen or vaccine.

Materials

*   Shaker incubator
*   Centrifuge
*   Water bath
*   Conical flask—250ml
*   Petri dish

*   Tryptone Soya Broth (Soybean casein digest medium)
*   Phosphate buffered saline (PBS) (see Appendix)

Procedure

1. A loopful of culture of *Aeromonas hydrophila* from the culture tube is streaked onto a Tryptone soya agar plate. The plate is incubated overnight at 37°C
2. From the streaked agar plate a single colony is inoculated into a Tryptone soya broth (900mg in 30ml double distilled water in 250ml conical flask) and incubated at 37°C overnight in shaker incubator.
3. The resulting *Aeromonas hydrophila* culture is heat killed at 60°C for 1 hour in a water bath (sterility can be checked by streaking on agar plate).
4. The heat-killed culture is centrifuged at 3000 rpm for 15 minutes.
5. The supernatant is discarded and the pellet is washed with PBS once.
6. The packed cells are resuspended in PBS to desired concentration – (for immunizing fish, 1x10^8 cells in 0.2 ml PBS).

C. Preparation of 1. Soluble protein antigen 2. Particulate protein antigen and 3. Adjuvant – soluble protein antigen emulsion (using Bovine Serum Albumin).

The protein antigen, Bovine Serum Albumin (BSA), is prepared in the soluble form or particulate form or emulsified with an adjuvant.

Materials

*   Beaker (10, 25 ml)
*   Syringes (2 or 5 ml),

*   Crystalline Bovine Serum Albumin (BSA),
*   Physiological saline (0.15 M) (see Appendix)
*   Freund's Complete Adjuvant (FCA)

- Freund's Incomplete Adjuvant (FIA) (containing paraffin oil and mannide mono–oleate)
- Refined coconut oil

Procedure

Soluble BSA

Soluble BSA (S-BSA) is prepared by overlaying the BSA powder (25mg/ml) on physiological saline (3ml) and allowing it to dissolve without agitation.

Heat-aggregated BSA

The particulate form of antigen, heat-aggregated BSA (HA-BSA) is prepared by heating the required concentration of S-BSA at 70°C for 5 minutes.

Adjuvant – BSA Emulsion

BSA – adjuvant emulsion is prepared by mixing equal volumes (1 ml each) of required concentrations of S-BSA and Freund's Complete or Incomplete Adjuvant or double refined coconut oil in a 10 or 25 ml beaker. The mixing is done effectively by rapid and repeated flushing of the mixture by a syringe (without needle) into beaker (10 or 25 ml beaker). The resultant emulsion should be a thick white solution (the quality of the emulsion can be confirmed by placing a small drop of it in water. When the drop stays intact and does not dissolve in the water, the emulsion is good and suitable for injection).

Freund's Complete Adjuvant (FCA) is widely used in research and is one of the first adjuvants developed. However, there are a number of significant disadvantages on its use. Freund's complete adjuvant causes local inflammatory lesions which can be quite severe and result in chronic granulomas, abscesses, and tissue sloughs. When injected into the footpad of an animal (say rabbit), it can cause chronic lameness and arthritis; injected intraperitoneally, it can cause peritonitis. Furthermore, accidental injection of FCA to the handling personnel can result in sensitization to tuberculin as well as chronic, local inflammation which is poorly responsive to antibiotic therapy. Therefore, alternative adjuvants should be considered.

References

1. Nakano, K., Studies on the role of macrophages in the antibody response of mice: the relationship between the immunogenicity of different forms of antigen and the mode of antigen handling by macrophages. J Reticuloendothel Soc, 1976. **19**(6): p. 361-74.
2. Logambal, S.M. and R.D. Michael, Immunostimulatory effect of azadirachtin in *Oreochromis mossambicus* (Peters). Indian Journal of Experimental Biology, 2000. **38**(11): p. 1092-1096.
3. Logambal, S.M., S. Venkatalakshmi, and R. Dinakaran Michael, Immunostimulatory effect of leaf extract of *Ocimum sanctum* Linn. in *Oreochromis mossambicus* (Peters). Hydrobiologia, 2000. 430(1-3): p. 113-120.
4. Karunasagar, I., A. Ali, and S. Otta, Immunization with bacterial antigens: infections with motile aeromonads. Developments in biological standardization, 1996. 90: p. 135-141.

5. Sailendri, K. and Muthukkaruppan, V.R., The immune response of the teleost, Tilapia mossambica to soluble and cellular antigens. Journal of Experimental Zoology, 1975. 191(3): p. 371-381.

.... **Notes/Records** ....

1.4 IMMUNIZATION

Introduction

Though fishes are the most primitive group among the vertebrates, they have primary and secondary lymphoid organs. Fishes can produce fairly good antibody response and they exhibit immunological memory with an enhanced secondary antibody response. However, there is no isotype switch and so both in the primary and secondary responses, they produce only tetramer IgM type immunoglobulin.

Materials

- Tilapia 50 – 100g (As per requirement)
- 1ml tuberculin Syringe & 24-gauge needle

- Bovine Serum Albumin (BSA)
- Saline (Physiological saline)
- FCA\FIA\purified coconut oil

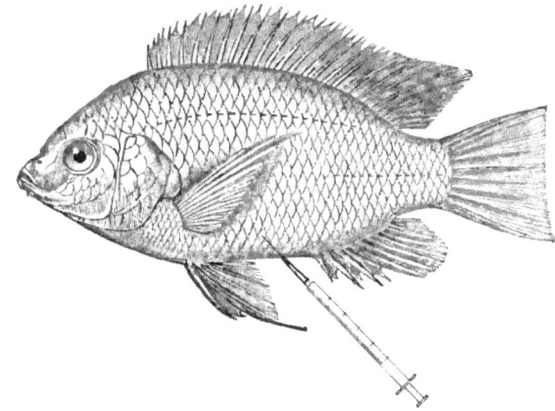

Figure 1.7 Site of intraperitoneal injection in fish.

Procedure

1. 25mg of BSA is weighed and dissolved in 1ml of saline in a 10 ml beaker.
2. To this, 1ml of adjuvant (FCA / FIA/coconut oil) is added and made into a milky white emulsion (by repeated suction and flushing using a syringe without needle) 0.4ml of the emulsion is injected intraperitoneally / intramuscularly in to fish.
3. Two weeks later, a booster dose (0.4 ml of BSA-Adjuvant emulsion) is given.
4. After 2 weeks, the fish are bled to get 0.1 ml to 0.2 ml blood.
5. Blood is transferred to a glass serology tube and allowed to clot for one hour at room temperature.
6. The clot is loosened from the sides of the tube to aid retraction.
7. For the serum to be expressed, it is left in the fridge at 4°C overnight.
8. After 24 hours, the serum is separated by centrifugation at 2000 rpm for 15 minutes and transferred to plastic storage vials. The harvested serum is likely to be a hyperimmune serum raised in the fish against BSA.

Note: Passive haemagglutination assay can be performed (refer relevant section in this manual) to find out the $\log_2$ antibody titre of the antiserum.

.... **Notes/Records** ....

1.5 REPETITIVE BLEEDING TECHNIQUE

Blood is drawn from animals for a variety of scientific purposes. Scientists should be aware that the process may be stressful for an animal, simply because of the handling, the type of anaesthetic used/not used or the pain/discomfort caused by a particular bleeding procedure. The physiological changes associated with increased stress may even invalidate the results. To raise polyclonal antiserum in an animal, there should be reliable methods available to repetitively bleed that animal. The blood thus collected is allowed to clot and the serum (which contains the polyclonal antibodies, hence called antiserum) can be separated from the clot normally by centrifugation. Repetitive bleeding method is always better than sacrificing the animal for many reasons including the possibility for test bleeding and for analysing the kinetics of antibody response in individual animals. Although bleeding is one of the common procedures performed on laboratory animals, care should be taken to minimize the stress (e.g. by anaesthetizing the animal) not only for ethical reasons but also for not altering the animal's physiological/immunological parameters after bleeding.

The volume of blood required and frequency of the requirement will determine the method and site of bleeding. Proper insertion of the needle into a vein or other part of the vascular system is normally the most critical part of the procedure. Certain guidelines can be given, but only practice provides proficiency. Veins may be expected to roll, collapse or shift, making insertion of needle difficult. A precise, careful introduction of the needle is the best and several attempts may be required. The needle is inserted parallel to the vein and the tip directed into the lumen along the longitudinal axis. When withdrawing blood from a vein, aspiration should be slow so that the vessel does not collapse.

Materials

- Tilapia weighing 50 g
- Alcohol (70% ethanol)

- Syringes (1 ml, 2 ml tuberculin)
- Pasteur pipette
- Suction tube
- Serology tube
- Cotton

Procedure

Common cardinal vein bleeding in fish (Michael et al., 1994)

1. The fish is held with right lateral side facing the investigator (the fish may be anaesthetized by keeping it in MS222 or 2-Phenoxyethanol (100 ppm) dissolved water, see appendix).
2. The right operculum and the gills are lifted using small metal rod or a lancet to expose the common cardinal vein.
3. The blood is drawn from the common cardinal vein using 1 ml tuberculin syringe with 24-gauge needle.

4. Easily about 0.1 to 0.3 ml blood can be drawn and transferred to small serology tube for clotting and serum separation.

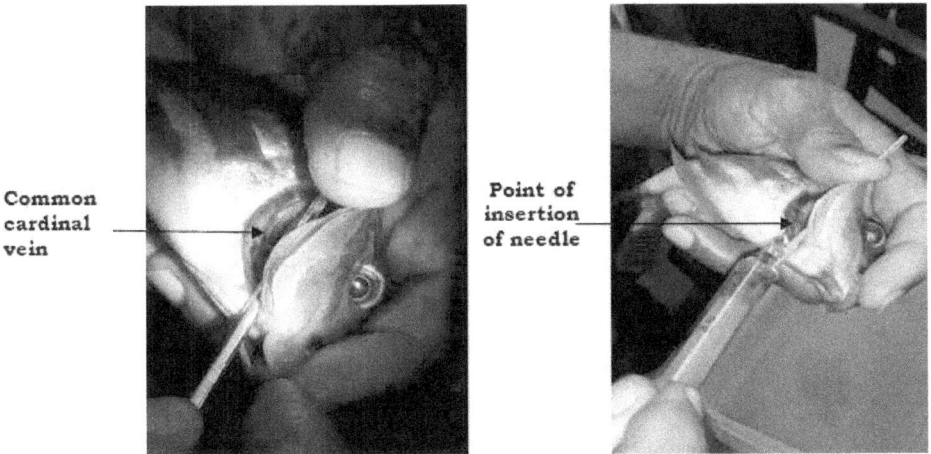

Figure 1.8 Location of common cardinal vein for repetitive bleeding.

References

1. A rapid method for repetitive bleeding in fish. Michael R.D., Srinivas S.D., Sailendri K., and V.R. Muthukkaruppan. Ind. J. Exp. Biol. 32: 838- 839, 1994.

2. Michael, R.D. and S.K. Priyadarshini, A reliable method for repetitive bleeding in striped murrel, *Channa striata* (Bloch). Aquaculture Research, 2012. 43(11): p. 1738.

.... **Notes/Records** ....

.... **Notes/Records** ....

2. VACCINES

INTRODUCTION

The word vaccine is derived from Latin, *Vacca* means cow. Edward Jenner is the pioneer in vaccine who in 1798 successfully developed vaccine against small pox using cow pox virus without actually knowing underlying immunological mechanisms. About a hundred years later, Louis Pasteur with his knowledge in Microbiology, successfully developed and demonstrated the basic mechanisms of vaccine and vaccination. By definition, vaccines are killed or attenuated microbial pathogens or their components or products which on administration to a host, make that host immune (resistant) to subsequent infection by naturally occurring corresponding (virulent) pathogen.

2.1 PREPARATION OF *A. HYDROPHILA* VACCINE AND EFFICACY TESTING

Principle

Vaccines are killed or attenuated microbial pathogens or their components or products which on administration to a host, make the host immune (resistant) to the natural infection by the corresponding pathogen. Large number of vaccines have been developed for humans and livestock. With the advent of intensive fish culture (due to the realization of the economic and nutritional value of fish) and the consequent disease problems in aquaculture, the fish immunologists have developed some vaccines to protect the fish form infectious diseases.

The principle of vaccines and vaccination is that when an animal is vaccinated, it produces antibody producing cells which mount primary antibody response. Some of the potential antibody producing cells develop into memory cells which will be circulating in the system. When the vaccinated animal is infected by the virulent naturally occurring pathogen (against which the animal is vaccinated) the specific memory cells on recognition of the pathogen, rapidly proliferate and produce large amount of antibodies to neutralize the pathogen and thus protect the animal from the infectious diseases.

The protective efficacy of a vaccine can be tested experimentally by performing a 'challenge' test. This test involves vaccinated fish and unvaccinated control fish. Some days after vaccination, both the groups of fish can be challenged (injected) with virulent pathogen and mortality of fish in both the groups can be recorded to calculate the relative percent survival by a simple formula which will reflect the efficacy of the developed vaccine.

Materials

- Colorimeter
- Orbital shaker incubator

- Centrifuge (50 mL tubes)
- Micropipettes
- Autoclavable Centrifuge Tubes
- Spectrophotometer
- Conical flasks
- Water Bath
- Syringes (1 ml, tuberculin)
- Biohazard waste disposal cover for collection of dead fish
- Facemask and powder free gynaecological gloves to handle fish.
- Test tubes

- Tilapia 40-50g (As per requirement)
- Virulent *Aeromonas hydrophila* strain with known LD_{50} value
- Soybean Casein Digest Medium
- Sterile phosphate buffered saline (PBS)
- Distilled Water
- Agar

Procedure

1. For vaccine preparation, overnight culture of virulent *A. hydrophila* in 30 ml soybean casein digest medium is kept in a water bath at 60 °C for 1 hour in order to completely kill all the bacteria.
2. Sterility of the preparation is checked by plating heat killed organism into fresh soybean casein digest agar and ensuring no colony formation.
3. Heat killed bacteria i.e. vaccine is then centrifuged at 3000 rpm for 10 min. The resulting supernatant is discarded and to the pellet, 30 ml sterile PBS is added.
4. Step 3 is repeated one more time and ensured that there is no retention of soybean casein digestion medium.
5. OD is measured using colorimeter at 490 nm and adjusted to 1.2. This preparation is now called as vaccine which may contain 5×10^8 cells/ml as standardized earlier in this laboratory.
6. The prepared vaccine (0.2 ml/fish) is then intra-peritoneally administered to a group of ten fish.
7. Another group (control) of ten fish are also injected intra-peritoneally with 0.2 ml sterile PBS each.
8. Fourteen days after vaccination, both the vaccinated and the control groups are challenged (administered) with LD_{50} dose (0.2 ml/fish) of virulent A.hydrophila by intra-peritoneal injection.
9. After challenge, record the cumulative mortality of fishes for 4 days.
10. Efficacy of vaccine can be determined in terms of relative per cent survival of the fish (RPS) which is calculated by the formula

$$\text{RPS} = \left\{ 1 - \frac{\text{Per cent mortality in treated group}}{\text{Per cent mortality in control group}} \right\} \times 100$$

References

1. Subramani, P. A., Daniels Gnanamuthu, A. A. and Michael, R. D. (2016), Neutrophil activity affects *Oreochromis mossambicus* (Peters, 1852) antibody production against heat-killed *Aeromonas hydrophila* vaccine. J. Appl. Ichthyol., 32: 1113–1117. doi:10.1111/jai.13123.

2. Chandran MR, Aruna BV, Logambal SM, Michael RD. Immunisation of Indian major carps against Aeromonas hydrophila by intraperitoneal injection. Fish Shellfish Immunol. 2002 Jul; 13(1):1-9.

.... **Notes/Records** ....

.... **Notes/Records** ....

3. SPECIFIC HUMORAL IMMUNE RESPONSE

Immunity in vertebrates is the host's defense against infection by pathogens, entry of other antigens and/or internally emerging malignancy or cancer. Immunity can be divided in non-specific or innate immunity and specific or acquired immunity. Non-specific or innate immune mechanisms which are always present (even in the absence of antigen) in the host and can work against all potential antigens. It is the first line of defense. On the other hand specific or acquired or adaptive immune responses which are elicited only after the entry of antigen and directed specifically against that entered antigen.

The specific immune responses are mediated by T and B cells following exposure to antigen and the responses are characterized by 'non self' recognition, specificity and immunological memory. Specific immunity is further divided into humoral immunity which is mediated by substances (antibodies) present in humors of the body (blood and lymph) and Cell mediated immunity mediated by T cells.

The Humoral Immune Response (HI) is the immune reaction that is mediated by secreted antibodies, produced by the cells of the B lymphocyte (B cell) lineage. Secreted antibodies bind to antigens (present on the surfaces of invading microbes such as viruses or bacteria), which ultimately results in their destruction.

All Mammals (e.g. mice, rabbits) produce pentamer IgM antibodies during the primary response and during secondary response, they produce IgG antibodies with the same antigenic specificity (Isotype switch). On the other hand, being a primitive vertebrate, fishes produce only tetramer IgM in both primary and secondary responses and hence there is no isotype switch in fishes.

Agglutination is a method by which the specific antibodies to cellular antigens present in polyclonal antiserum are quantified. The word agglutination comes from the Latin word *agglutinare*, meaning 'to glue to' Agglutinins are antibodies that produce agglutination, a reaction that occurs when the specific antibodies bind to antigenic determinants (epitopes) present on the surface of cellular antigens. The results of such a cross linking reaction are visible because of the formation of lattice or mesh. The lattices are composed of antibodies bridging or cross-linking the cellular antigens (or indicator cells coated with soluble antigens and their specific antibodies). This method is reliable and fairly sensitive.

3.1   HAEMAGGLUTINATION ASSAY

Introduction

Haemagglutination is an agglutination that involves red blood cells as antigens. It is the agglutination of red blood cells by specific antibodies directed against the antigens present on cell surface of red blood cells.

Principle

When specific antibodies react with antigenic epitopes on red blood cells (RBCs), they can cause cross linking of the RBCs resulting in agglutination or 'clumping together' of the cells. The minimum quantity of antibodies required for the agglutination RBCs provided, is expressed as the antibody titre of the antiserum.

Materials

- Microtitre plate (96 well "V" bottom)
- Micropipette – 50µl range
- Micropipette tips

- Physiological saline (0.15M) (see Appendix)
- 1% SRBC in physiological saline
- Anti-serum samples (at least 50µl/sample)

Procedure

1. The antigen (1% SRBC in saline) is prepared.
2. Fifty microlitre of physiological saline is added using a dropper or micropippette to all the wells of a clean 96 well 'V' bottom microtitre plate.
3. Fifty microlitre of the antiserum (anti-SRBC) is added in the first well, mixed well and 50 µl of this diluted serum is taken and added to the next well and so on thus serially double diluting in the wells of the first row up to the 11th well. The 12th well is left (without any addition of serum) as the negative control.
4. Similarly, other serum samples are also diluted serially in the other rows of the microtitre plate.
5. Twenty-five microlitre of the antigen (1% SRBC/HRBC) is added to all the wells of the microtitre plate.
6. The microtitre plate is gently hand-shaken for efficient mixing of the reagents.
7. The plate is incubated at room temperature for an hour.
8. The highest dilution of the serum samples which shows detectable agglutination (lattice-mat formation) is recorded and expressed as $\log_2$ antibody titre of the serum.

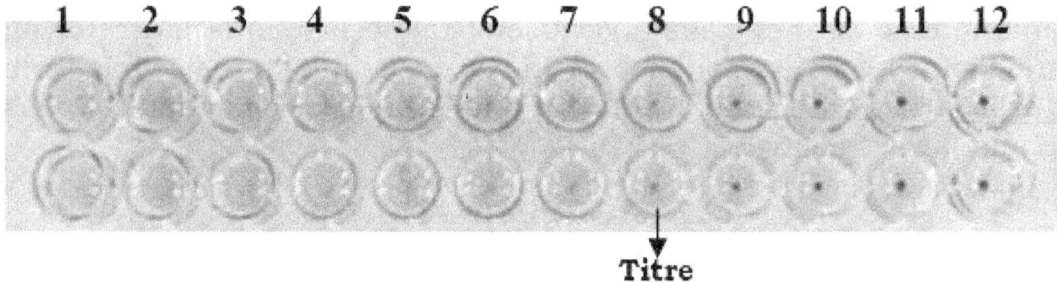

Figure 3.1   Haemagglutination (note: In some laboratories, the well showing more than 50% mat formation is considered as $\log_2$ antibody titre, in this case-8).

References

1. Sailendri, K. and Muthukkaruppan, V.R., The immune response of the teleost, Tilapia mossambica to soluble and cellular antigens. Journal of Experimental Zoology, 1975. 191(3): p. 371-381.

2. Logambal, S.M. and R.D. Michael, Immunostimulatory effect of azadirachtin in *Oreochromis mossambicus* (Peters). Indian Journal of Experimental Biology, 2000. **38**(11): p. 1092-1096.

3. Logambal, S.M., S. Venkatalakshmi, and R. Dinakaran Michael, Immunostimulatory effect of leaf extract of *Ocimum sanctum* Linn. in *Oreochromis mossambicus* (Peters). Hydrobiologia, 2000. 430(1-3): p. 113-120.

.... **Notes/Records** ....

3.2 PASSIVE AGGLUTINATION ASSAY

Introduction

Passive Agglutination assay is the test to quantify the antibodies against soluble antigens using the principle of agglutination. The passive agglutination is much more sensitive than direct agglutination. Here the antibody titre is determined by the agglutination of red blood cells coated with a soluble antigen (e.g bovine serum albumin-BSA) by specific antibodies directed against BSA (coated on to the red cells). The indicator cells used for this assay can be RBCs or any other substances suitable for agglutination like latex beads or even gold particles.

Principle

In this technique, antigen-coated red blood cells are prepared by coupling a soluble antigen (BSA) with sheep red blood cells (indicator cells) using chromic chloride as the coupling agent. When the BSA coated sheep red blood cells are mixed with specific anti-BSA antiserum, cross-linking and agglutination of coated erythrocytes occur by specific antibodies binding with the antigenic determinants of BSA coated onto the erythrocytes.

Materials

- Microtitre plate (96 well "V" bottom)
- Micropipette – 50 µl
- Micropipette tips
- Glass pipette 1ml
- Beaker 10ml
- Conical flask – 25ml, 50ml
- Glass centrifuge tubes-15ml

- Physiological saline (0.15M) (see appendix)
- Bovine Serum Albumin (BSA)
- Chromic chloride
- Sheep red blood cells in Alsever's solution
- Antiserum samples

Procedure

A. Coupling BSA to SRBC (Michael, 1986)

1. Chromic chloride is an effective coupling agent for linking proteins to red blood cells.
2. Sheep red blood cells in Alsever's solution are washed **thrice** with physiological saline (0.15N) by centrifuging every time at 3000 rpm for 10 minutes.
3. To one volume of packed SRBC (say, 0.5ml) equal volumes of BSA at a concentration of 5mg/ml saline and equal volume of chromic chloride solution at a concentration of 1mg/1ml saline are added.
4. The mixture is agitated by hand for 10 minutes and kept in a water bath at 37°C for 15 minutes with intermittent agitation.
5. The reaction is stopped abruptly by diluting with saline.

6. The BSA coupled cells are washed thrice in saline and resuspended to the required concentration in saline. Normally 1% BSA – coated SRBC is used for antibody titration.

B. Antibody titration

1. Fifty microlitre of physiological saline is added (0.15N) (using a micropipette) to each well in the microtitre plate.
2. To this, 50μl of antiserum is added to the first well in a row and a two-fold serial dilution is made in the wells of the first row till the 11th well of the microtitre plate, leaving the 12th well as negative control.
3. Then 50μl (or 25μl) of 1% BSA coupled SRBC in saline is added to all the wells.
4. The microtitre plate is hand- shaken for effective mixing of reagents.
5. The reagents are incubated for an hour at 37°C and for more hours at 10°C.
6. The highest dilution of the serum samples which shows detectable (mat formation) agglutination is recorded and expressed as $\log_2$ antibody titre of the serum.

References

1. Jandl, J.H. and R.L. Simmons, The agglutination and sensitization of red cells by metallic cations: interactions between multivalent metals and the red-cell membrane. Br J Haematol, 1957. **3**(1): p. 19-38.
2. Michael, R.D., Studies on the immune response to BSA in the lizard, *Calotes versicolor.*, in Zoology1986, Ph.D. thesis, Madurai Kamaraj University: TN, India.
3. Michael RD, Priscilla AS. Diel variations in antibody response to bovine serum albumin in *Oreochromis mossambicus* (Peters). Indian J Exp Biol. 1994 Jul; 32(7):474-7.
4. Muthulakshmi M, Subramani PA, Michael RD. Immunostimulatory effect of the aqueous leaf extract of *Phyllanthus niruri* on the specific and nonspecific immune responses of *Oreochromis mossambicus* Peters. Iran J Vet Res. 2016 Summer; 17(3):200-202.

.... **Notes/Records** ....

.... **Notes/Records** ....

3.3   BACTERIAL AGGLUTINATION ASSAY

Introduction

Agglutination reactions are among the most easily performed immunological tests. A bacterial infection often elicits the production of serum antibodies specific for surface antigens of the bacterial cells. The presence of such antibodies can be detected by bacterial agglutination assays. Many bacterial species form smooth suspensions in buffered saline. When incubated with antibodies directed against surface antigens like those of flagella, capsular material or cell wall components, the bacteria are agglutinated to form clumps. The agglutination is due to cross linking of cellular (bacterial) antigens by bivalent or multivalent antibodies. This method, though semi quantitative, is reliable and fairly sensitive.

Principle

The specific antibodies present in antiserum raised against cellular bacterial antigen (e.g. *Aeromonas hydrophila*) when react with the specific antigenic epitopes on the bacteria, cause agglutination or clumping together of the bacteria. The result of such a cross linking reaction is visible because of the formation of lattice or mesh. The lattice is composed of multi valent antibodies cross-linking the bacterial antigens. The minimum quantity of antibodies required for (or maximum diluted antiserum which can cause) visible agglutination is expressed as the antibody titre of the antiserum.

Materials

- Centrifuge
- Incubator
- Colorimeter
- Water bath
- 96 well "V" bottom microtitre plate
- Conical flasks
- Pipette (range 5-50µl, 20-200µl)

- *Aeromonas hydrophila* (overnight culture).
- Normal and antiAh antiserum
- Tryptic soy broth
- Phosphate Buffered Saline (PBS) (see appendix)
- Crystal violet stain

Procedure

1. Twenty-five microlitre of PBS is added using a 25 µl micropipette into all the wells of a clean "V-bottom" microtitre plate.
2. Twenty-five microlitre of antiserum is added to the first well and serially double diluted in that row of the plate till the 11ᵗʰ well leaving the 12ᵗʰ well as negative control in a 96 well microtitre plate.

3. To this, 25µl of heat killed pre-stained bacterial antigen (10^9 cells per ml) is added to all the wells.

4. The microtitre plates are mildly shaken for effective mixing of the reagents and then covered with a plastic film or cover.

5. The plates are incubated for overnight at 37°C

6. The highest dilution of the serum sample that shows detectable agglutination (macroscopic) is recorded and expressed as $\log_2$ antibody titre of the serum.

Note: A day before carrying out the assay, a single colony of *A. hydrophila* is inoculated into tryptone soya broth and incubated at 37°C overnight in shaker. Then the overnight culture is heat killed at 60°C for 1 hour in a water bath. The heat killed culture is washed thrice with PBS and centrifuged at 3000 rpm for 15 min. The packed cells are resuspended to desired concentration (say, 10^9 cells/ml) with PBS and stained with appropriate amount of Crystal Violet stain (about 200µl of CV /100 ml culture).

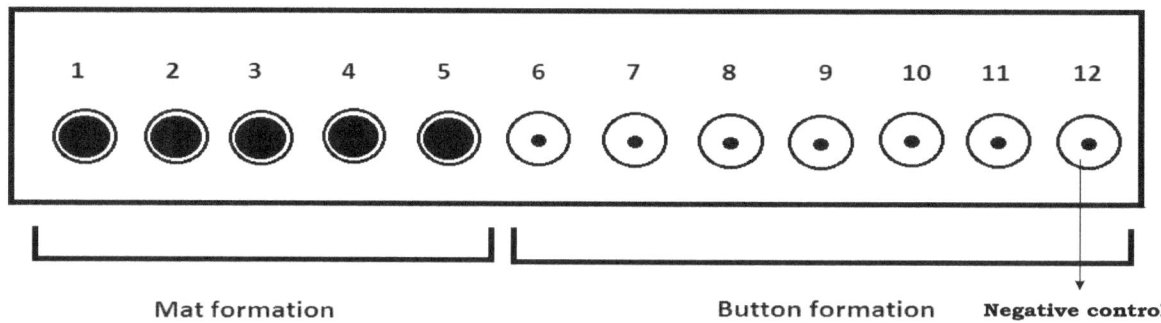

Figure 3.2 Diagrammatic representation of typical bacterial agglutination and button formation.

References

1. Karunasagar, I., A. Ali, and S. Otta, Immunization with bacterial antigens: infections with motile aeromonads. Developments in biological standardization, 1996. **90**: p. 135-141.

2. Kirubakaran CJ, Subramani PA, Michael RD. Methanol extract of *Nyctanthes arbortristis* seeds enhances non-specific immune responses and protects *Oreochromis mossambicus* (Peters) against *Aeromonas hydrophila* infection. Res Vet Sci. 2016 Apr; 105:243-8. doi: 10.1016/j.rvsc.2016.02.013.

3. Sudhakaran DS, Srirekha P, Devasree LD, Premsingh S, Michael RD. Immunostimulatory effect of *Tinospora cordifolia* Miers leaf extract in *Oreochromis mossambicus*. Indian J Exp Biol. 2006 Sep; 44(9):726-32.

.... **Notes/Records** ....

3.4 ENZYME LINKED IMMUNOSORBENT ASSAY (ELISA)

Introduction

Enzyme Linked Immunosorbent Assay also called by its acronym 'ELISA' is a biochemical technique used mainly in immunology to detect and quantify the specific antibody or an antigen in a sample. ELISA technique was conceptualized and developed by Peter Perlmann and Eva Engvall at Stockholm University, Sweden, in 1971 who demonstrated quantitative measurement of IgG in rabbit serum with alkaline phosphatase as the 'reporter' label. ELISA is based on the principle of immunoassay including that of enzyme-substrate reaction. ELISA has become extraordinarily useful because it allows rapid screening or quantitation of multiple samples for the presence of an antigen or the antibody. ELISA also remains very popular because of its specificity, sensitivity, reliability and ease of performance by automation and the ready availability of commercial labelled antibody reagents.

Principle

In ELISA, the antigen or antibody is attached to a solid phase (e.g. microtiter plate wells). Then the test sample (containing the specific antigen or antibody) is added to the wells. If the reagents are complementary to each other, the molecules (antigen or antibody) in the test sample will get attached to the complementary molecules in the wells. The antigen-antibody complex thus formed, can be visualized by treating with a second antibody conjugated/labelled with an enzyme and then added with the substrate. The colour developed is proportional to the concentration of the enzyme-labelled second antibody which in turn proportional to the concentration of Ab/Ag in the test sample.

Materials

- Microplate reader [Bio-Rad, USA]
- Microtitre plate (96 well flat bottom) [ELISA Plates, Greiner, Germany]

- Primary antibody (test sample from fish)
- Secondary antibody: Rabbit anti fish IgM,
- Tertiary antibody conjugated with an enzyme: Goat anti rabbit IgG-HRP conjugate, [Sigma, USA]
- Overnight *Aeromonas hydrophila* culture

Coating Buffer: Phosphate Buffered Saline (PBS) (see appendix)

Sodium chloride (0.15M)

Carbonate bicarbonate buffer (pH 9.6) (see appendix)

Blocking agent: Bovine serum Albumin [BSA - fraction V, Sigma, USA]

Substrate: 3, 3, 5, 5' Tetramethylbenzidine - Hydrogen Peroxide (TMB –H_2O_2), [Genei, Bangalore].

Reaction stop solution: 2N Sulphuric acid

Wash solution: Phosphate buffered saline – Tween 20 (polyoxyethylenesorbitan monolaurate) solution, pH 7.2 (PBS-T: 0.05% of Tween-20 is added to the Phosphate Buffer Saline)

Reagents Preparation

- Wash Solution (PBS-T Phosphate buffered saline – Tween), pH 7.2 (PBS-T)
- NaCl   8.00g
- KCl   0.20g
- $Na_2HPO_4.12H_2O$ 1.33g
- Tween 20   0.5ml
- Distilled water   1L
- Saline (Sodium chloride, 0.15M)
- Sodium chloride 0.87g
- Distilled water 1L
- 0.05M Sodium citrate buffer, pH 4.2
- Sodium citrate 14.70g
- Distilled water 1L

Procedure

1. Overnight culture of *A. hydrophila* is centrifuged at 3000 rpm for 15 min, washed twice with 0.15M NaCl solution and adjusted to 5×10^7 cells ml^{-1} in carbonate bicarbonate buffer.
2. Flat bottomed, 96-well microtitre (ELISA) plates are coated with 100 µl of the bacterial suspension of above mentioned concentration. The ELISA plates are incubated for 1 h at 37°C (or overnight at 4°C).
3. Then the plates are washed thrice with PBS-T
4. After that, 100 µl of 1% BSA in PBS is added to all the wells to block the unbound spaces (to prevent nonspecific adsorption of sample serum components) and the plates were incubated for 1 h at 37°C.
5. Then the plates are washed thrice with PBS-T
6. One hundred microlitre of test serum samples (1:10 or appropriately diluted) are added and the plates are incubated for 1 hr at 37°C (this temperature is found to be the optimum for tilapia antiserum)
7. The plates are washed thrice with PBS-T
8. After washing, 100 µl of polyclonal rabbit anti-fish IgM (1:100 or appropriately diluted) is added and the plates are incubated for 1 hr at room temperature, and then washed thrice with PBS-T.
9. One hundred microlitre of horse radish peroxidase (HRP)-conjugated goat anti-rabbit IgG at a dilution of 1:2000 (or appropriated) is added and the plates are incubated for 1 hr at room temperature.
10. Decant the supernatant and the plates are washed thrice with PBS-T and then 100µl of substrate solution (TMB-H_2O_2) is added.
11. The plates are left for 5 min for reaction and consequent colour development and the reaction is stopped by adding 25 µl of 1N sulphuric acid.

12. The optical density of plates is measured at 450 nm using an ELISA plate reader (Bio-Rad, USA).

Note: O.D value twice or more of negative control O.D can be taken as positive.

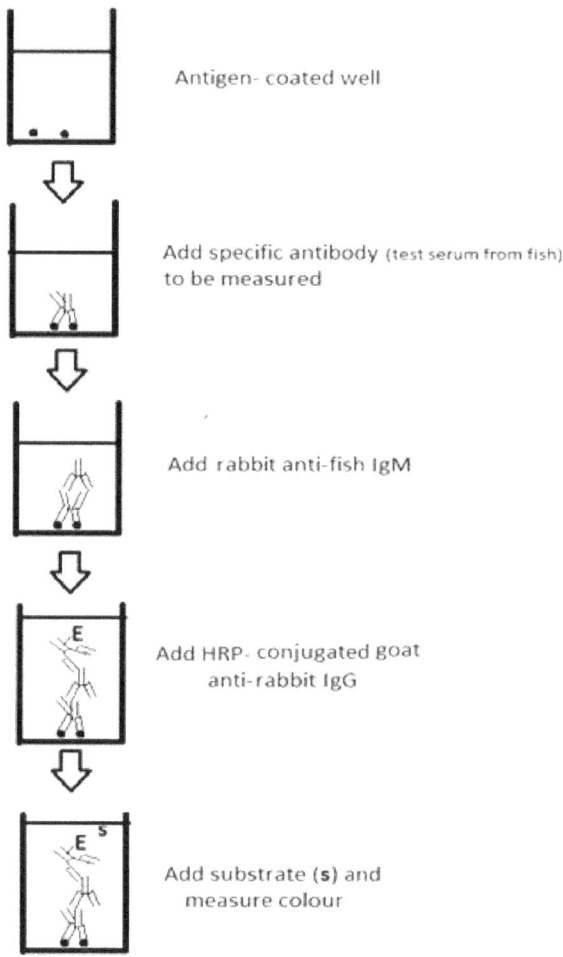

Figure 3.3   Diagrammatic representation of Enzyme-Linked Immunosorbent Assay

References

1.   Delamare, A.P.L., Echeverrigaray, S., Duarte, K.R., Gomes, L.H., Costa, S.O.P. Production of a monoclonal antibody against *Aeromonas hydrophila* and its application to bacterial identification. J. Appl. Microbiol. 2002 92:936–940.

2.   Kettman, J. & Wetzel, M. Antibody synthesis in vitro marker of B-cell differentiation. Journal of Immunological Methods 1980 39: 203.

3.   Binuramesh C, Prabakaran M, Steinhagen D, Michael RD. Effect of sex ratio on the immune system of *Oreochromis mossambicus* (Peters). Brain Behav Immun. 2006 May; 20(3):300-8.

.... **Notes/Records** ....

3.5 PLAQUE FORMING CELL ASSAY

Introduction

Plaque forming cell (PFC) assay is a quantitative technique used for enumerating the number of antigen specific antibody (IgM) producing cells present in a particular lymphoid organ (Ladics, 2005). For this assay, SRBC and spleen were conventionally used as the antigen and the lymphoid organ of choice respectively. The principle of this assay is actually derived from plaque-forming unit assay used to enumerate virus particles.

Principle

When antibody producing cells with membrane bound anti SRBC antibodies (IgM) encounters SRBC in the assay condition, antibody-SRBC complexes are formed. Upon addition of freshly prepared complement (usually from Guinea pig complement [serum], or freshly prepared fish homologous serum (from the fish species of the anti-SRBC antibody source), results in complement mediated lysis of SRBC leading to the formation of clear area/zone (termed as plaque) around the antibody producing cell. The assay is conducted in a semisolid agar gels containing SRBC and the plaques (equal to number of antibody producing cells) per volume of sample are enumerated and can be calculated for the entire lymphoid organ (spleen).

Materials

- 2 ml syringes with 24G needles
- Microscope slides (Preferably with scratched or agar pre-coated surface)
- Micropipette – 50 µl
- Micropipette tips
- Microscope
- Disposable cell strainer– 100 µm mesh fitted on 15-ml centrifuge tubes
- Refrigerated centrifuge
- Serological tubes
- Neubauer's chamber

- Tilapia 40-50g (number as per requirement)
- Phenoxy ethanol/ or any other recommended anaesthetic
- SRBC
- Sterile phosphate buffered saline (PBS)
- Distilled Water
- Agarose (low melting point)
- RPMI-1640 media
- Guinea pig serum or homologous tilapia serum

Procedure

1. Fish are injected i.p. with 0.1ml of 5% SRBC. After 3 days, a booster dose of 0.1ml of 25% SRBC is administered i.p.

2. Ten days after injecting SRBC, the fish are sacrificed using overdose of phenoxy ethanol and the spleen is aseptically excised.

3. The spleen is placed over the cell strainer (fitted on 15 ml centrifuge tubes) and gently pressed using sterile glass pestle (or a glass plunger of 1ml syringe) and 2-3 ml RPMI-1640 medium is added to flush the cells into the centrifuge tubes.

4. This cell suspension is washed twice with RPMI-1640 by centrifuging (400xg).

5. The cell suspension is adjusted with RPMI-1640 to contain $1x10^7$cells/ml.

6. One hundred microlitres of cell suspension, 200 µl of 10% SRBC, 100 µl of 1.5% solution of warm agarose (45°C) and 100 µl of RPMI 1640 are mixed in a serology tube and quickly poured onto a glass slide with scratched or pre-coated* surface (for adherence of agarose to the slide) and incubated for 4 h at 28°C.

7. Then freshly prepared 500 µl of 10% guinea pig serum or homologous tilapia serum (complement source) is added to the slide and further incubated for 2 h at 28°C.

8. The number of visible plaques per slide is then enumerated (Anderson, 1990) using a binocular microscope with a low magnification.

9. From the dilution (factor) of cell suspension to have $1x10^7$cells/ml and cell sample volume (100 µl) on the glass slide, total number of antibody producing cells in the spleen of a fish can be calculated.

*Pre-coating makes the surface of glass slide to adhere firmly to agar/agarose gel and also prevent capillary leakage of reagents between glass and agar surface. Pre-coating is done either by coating the slide with a thin layer of 0.2 - 0.5% agar by adding about 0.5 ml to cover entire surface or by brushing the hot agar solution on to the surface of a slide using a brush or cotton or gauze and drying the coated slide in a hot air oven for a minutes.

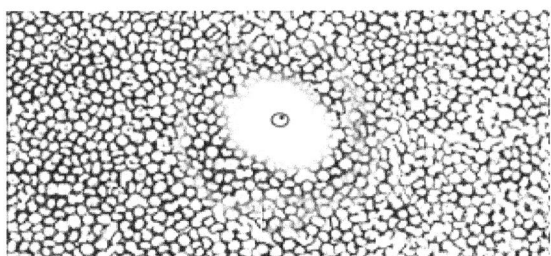

Figure 3.4   A plaque with an antibody producing (or plaque forming) cell in the centre surrounded by unaffected sheep erythrocytes

References

1. Sailendri, K. and Muthukkaruppan, V.R., The immune response of the teleost, Tilapia mossambica to soluble and cellular antigens. Journal of Experimental Zoology, 1975. 191(3):371-381.

2. Ladics, G. Plaque-Forming Cell Assays. Encyclopaedia of Immunotoxicology. H.-W. Vohr. Berlin, Heidelberg, Springer Berlin Heidelberg: 2005. 1-5.

3. Logambal SM, Venkatalakshmi S, Dinakaran Michael R. Immunostimulatory effect of leaf extract of *Ocimum sanctum* Linn. in *Oreochromis mossambicus* (Peters). Hydrobiologia. 2000; 430 (1):113-20.

4. Anderson, D.P. Passive haemolytic plaque assay for detecting antibody producing cells in fish. In: Stolen, J.S., Fletcher, T.C., Anderson, D.P., Roberson, B.S., Van Muiswinkel, W.B. (Eds.), Techniques in Fish Immunology. SOS Publications, New Jersey, 1990. pp. 9–12.

5. Binuramesh, C, Prabakaran, M, Steinhagen, D, Michael, RD. Effect of chronic confinement stress on the immune responses in different sex ratio groups of Oreochromis mossambicus (Peters). Aquaculture 250 (2005) 47– 59.

.... **Notes/Records** ....

4. IMMUNOGLOBULINS

Immunoglobulins are the antibodies secreted by plasma cells of B lymphocyte lineage. The immunoglobulins are the effector molecules of specific humoral immunity. They bind with the antigens that enter host and ultimately removed from the host system. In mammals the immunoglobulins are of five different classes, each with different kinds of structures and functions. Being primitive, the fishes mainly have only one type of immunoglobulins and they are of tetramer IgM type though monomer type of Immunoglobulins in mucus were also reported recently.

4.1 ISOLATION OF IMMUNOGLOBULIN FROM SERUM

Principle

The relative solubility of proteins in various salt solutions is used as the basic fractionation principle to separate the proteins. Ammonium sulphate precipitation is widely used for the preparation of an immunoglobulin fraction from whole serum. The use of ammonium sulphate rather than sodium sulphate as the precipitating salt offers the advantage of a high solubility of the former. Usually three precipitations are enough to separate Ig in a fairly pure form at a final ammonium sulphate concentration of 40% saturation.

Materials

- pH meter
- Magnetic stirrer
- Refrigerated /Cooling Centrifuge
- Beakers (10ml and other volume beakers)
- Graduated centrifuge tube
- Micropipettes
- Serological tubes
- Dialysis membrane-60 (Hi Media)
- Glass rod
- Twine/ holder

- Serum samples
- Ammonium sulphate (100% saturated pH 7.2)
- 40% Ammonium sulphate solution
- PBS
- EDTA
- Sodium bicarbonate
- Double distilled water

Procedure

1. One ml of serum is taken in a 10 ml beaker and diluted with 1ml PBS. To this 2ml diluted serum, 1.64ml of (100% saturated) ammonium sulphate solution is added **very slowly** (drop by drop). The ammonium sulphate concentration in this 3.64ml mixture is 45%.

2. Then the mixture is kept in an icebox (at 4°C) for 30 minutes during which the mixture is mildly shaken intermittently. At the end of 30 minutes, a cloudy white precipitate can be observed.

3. The precipitate is centrifuged at 2500 rpm for 15 min. The supernatant is discarded (first precipitation).

4. The pellet is washed with 1.64 ml of ammonium sulphate solution (100% saturated) and re-centrifuged at 2500 rpm for 15 minutes. The supernatant is discarded.

5. The pellet is re-dissolved gently in 1 ml of PBS and centrifuged at 2500 rpm for 10 min.

6. The pellet is discarded and the supernatant (1ml) is mixed with 0.67 ml of 100% saturated ammonium sulphate solution to achieve a 40% ammonium sulphate solution.

7. The precipitate formed is centrifuged (2500 rpm for 10 min) and the supernatant is discarded. The precipitate is washed with one ml (volume equal to the volume of serum originally used for precipitation) of 40% ammonium sulphate solution (second precipitation).

8. After centrifuging, the supernatant is discarded. The precipitate is mixed with minimum volume of PBS (less than 1ml). The sample is then dialysed with PBS with five changes at 4 °C, as mentioned below.

Dialysis

Dialysis is a method used to concentrate the immunoglobulins after ammonium sulphate fractionation or precipitation.

1. Initially 5mM of EDTA (1.86 mg/ml) and 20mM of Sodium bicarbonate (1.68 mg/ml) are dissolved in 100ml of distilled water in a 200ml beaker. The solution is heated to boil (flame/hot plate).

2. About 5 cm length of the dialysis bag (Dialysis membrane – 60, Hi Media, India) is kept in the above boiling solution for 5 minutes. This activates the dialysis membrane.

3. With the help of forceps, the dialysis bag is taken out and washed in distilled water.

4. One end of the dialysis bag is tied with twine (before use the twine is kept in the boiling distilled water for few minutes). Through the open end of the dialysis bag, the sample to be dialysed is quickly loaded. After loading the open end is also tied with twine.

5. The twine from both the ends is tied to a glass rod, which is kept on the beaker containing PBS (so that the dialysis bag is hanging and completely immersed in the PBS).

6. This beaker is kept on a mini magnetic stirrer and kept in a refrigerator (8 °C) for a period of 12 hours, with 5 changes of PBS at regular intervals, with slow, constant stirring using a small magnetic bar (care should be taken not be disturb the dialysis bag, while subjected to stirring).

7. After dialysis, the enriched immunoglobulin is frozen and stored for future use.

Confirmation of Immunoglobulin

Prepare a 1:20 dilution of sample and determine the peak absorbance using UV-VIS spectrophotometer. Immunoglobulins show maximal absorbance at 280 nm.

.... **Notes/Records** ....

4.2 QUANTIFICATION OF IMMUNOGLOBULIN

Introduction

Serum proteins (about 8% in blood) mainly include albumins, globulins and fibrinogens. Albumin is formed in the liver. Approximately 50-60 % of total serum protein is albumin, the rest is globulins. Albumin helps to maintain normal distribution of water in the body (colloidal osmotic pressure), and helps in the transport of blood constituents such as ions, pigments, bilirubin, hormones, enzymes and even the drugs we take. Globulin fraction contains gamma globulins (which are immunologically active hence, called immunoglobulins). The ratio of albumin to globulin is an important indicator of certain disease states. The total protein content in serum is measured following the method of Lowry *et al.* (1951). Albumin is measured by the Bromocresol Green method (Doumas, 1971). The globulin fraction is calculated by subtracting the albumin value from total protein value.

Estimation of Total Protein by Lowry Method

Principle

This is the most widely used method for quantitative determination of protein concentration. Reaction of the phenolic moiety of tyrosine (and other aromatic amino acids) in protein with Folin-Ciocalteau reagent, which contains phosphomolybdic/ tungstic acid mixture, produces a blue/purple colour with absorption maximum around 660 nm. Additionally, the use of copper reagent enhances the colour formation by chelating with peptide bonds and allowing efficient electron transfer to the chromophore formed. This method is sensitive down to 10 mg/ml protein.

Materials

- ELISA plate reader
- 96 well flat bottom microtitre plates
- Micropipettes

- Serum
- Saline
- Sodium tartrate
- Copper sulphate
- Sodium carbonate
- Sodium hydroxide
- Folin-Ciocalteau reagent (Commercially available)
- Bovine serum albumin (5mg/ml of saline)

Preparation of reagent A

- Sodium Potassium tartrate 20 mg
- Copper sulphate 10 mg
- Sodium carbonate 1 gm
- Sodium hydroxide 200 mg
- Distilled water 100 ml

- Reagent A1 -Dissolve Sodium Potassium tartrate in 1 ml distilled water
- Reagent A2 -Dissolve Copper sulphate in 1 ml distilled water
- Reagent A3 -Dissolve sodium carbonate in 50 ml of 0.1N sodium hydroxide

Reagent A

- Mix 500 µl of reagent A1, 500 µl of reagent A2 and 50 ml of A3 just before use.

Table 4.1 Preparation of protein (BSA) standard

S. No	Saline (µl)	BSA (stock solution 5mg/ml) (µl)	Amount of BSA (µg) in 400 µl saline	Final Concentration of BSA (µg/ml)
1	380	20	100	250
2	360	40	200	500
3	340	60	300	750
4	300	100	500	1250
5	200	200	1000	2500
6	100	300	1500	3750
7	-	400	2000	5000

Procedure

1. Ten microlitre of sample serum is diluted with 30 µl of saline in a well of 96 well flat bottom microtitre plates.
2. Forty microlitre of each BSA standard prepared (See Table above) are added to different wells of a row.
3. To this 200 µl of reagent A is added and incubated for 10 minutes at room temperature.
4. This mixture is reduced by 20 µl of Folin Phenol reagent and incubated for 30 minutes at room temperature and a blue colour is developed.
5. The optical density is read at 490 nm in a plate reader. Total protein is estimated from a standard curve prepared using bovine serum albumin.

***Note*:** For laboratory class room purposes, instead of plotting the standard graph (BSA) along with the test protein samples every time, the standard graph can be plotted once and test protein concentrations (of different samples at different times) can be directly read from the graph.

Estimation of Albumin

Principle

When the anionic bromocresol green reacts with albumin (by means of electrostatic forces, tertiary Vander Waal's forces and hydrogen bonding) at pH 4.2, it leads to a formation of a blue-green complex, the intensity of which is directly proportional to the albumin concentration of the serum.

Materials

- ELISA plate reader
- 96 well flat bottom microtitre plates
- Micropipettes

- Serum
- Succinate buffer
- Bromocresol green
- Brij
- Bovine Serum Albumin (5mg/ml of succinate buffer)

Bromocresol green stock solution

- Bromocresol green sodium salt 43.2 mg
- Sodium azide 10 mg
- Distilled water 100 ml
- Dissolve the reagents in distilled water and store in dark.

Working dye solution (pH 4.2)

- Bromocresol green stock solution 12 ml
- Succinate buffer 24 ml
- 30% Brij 35 200 µl
- Mix the three solutions just before use.

Table 4.2 Preparation of albumin standard

S. No	Succinate Buffer (µl)	BSA (stock solution 5mg/ml) (µl)	Amount of BSA (µg) in 50 µl solution	Final Concentration of BSA (µg/ml)
1	48	2	10	200
2	45	5	25	500
3	40	10	50	1000
4	35	15	75	1500
5	30	20	100	2000
6	25	25	125	2500
7	10	40	200	4000

Procedure

1. Ten microlitre of serum is diluted with 40 µl of succinate buffer.
2. Fifty microlitre of albumin standards (see Table above) were added to different wells.
3. To this 150 µl of working dye solution is added.
4. This mixture is incubated for 2 minutes at room temperature.

5. The optical density is read at 630 nm in a plate reader.
6. The quantity of albumin is read from the standard curve prepared earlier using bovine serum albumin.

Note: For laboratory class room purposes, instead of plotting the standard graph (BSA) along with the test albumin samples every time, the standard graph can be plotted once and the tested albumin concentrations (of different samples at different times) can be directly read from the graph.

References

1. Lowry, O. H.; Rosebrough, N. J.; Farr, A. L.; Randall, R. J. Protein measurement with the Folin phenol reagent. Jour. Biol. Chem. 1951. 193 (1): 265–75.
2. McPherson, I.G. & Everard, D.W. Serum albumin estimation: Modification of the bromocresol green method. Clinica Chimica Acta. 1972. 37: 117-121.

.... **Notes/Records** ....

.... **Notes/Records** ....

5. ANTIGEN-ANTIBODY INTERACTION

The primary interaction is the binding of antibody with antigen which is governed by two factors, affinity and avidity. Affinity is the combined strength (binding energy) of non covalent interactions between a single antigen binding site on an antibody molecule and a single antigenic epitope in an antigen and it is the affinity of the antibody for that epitope.

Avidity is the strength (binding energy) of multiple interactions between a multivalent antibody and a multivalent antigen. 'Avidity' implies the stability of antigen-antibody complex. The forces of primary interaction are monovalent and they are electrostatic/ionic, hydrogen bonding, hydrophobic and Vander Waal forces. All these forces require a very close proximity between the molecules. The primary interaction of antibody and antigen will result in secondary phenomena like precipitation and agglutination if there is a cross linking of multivalent antigen by antibodies which are at least divalent.

5.1 OUCHTERLONY DOUBLE IMMUNODIFFUSION

Introduction

Ouchterlony double immunodiffusion (ODD) test was developed by Örjan Ouchterlony, a Swedish immunologist in 1949. ODD is a simple method for qualitative analysis of antibody or antigen. The binding of an antibody to an antigen is the first and fundamental immunological reaction. Antibodies and soluble antigens (like proteins) form complexes that may ultimately result in the formation of a visible white aggregate called precipitate and the process, the precipitation. ODD is used to compare different antigen preparations and check the specificity of a polyclonal antiserum and compare the immunological similarity/identity among the antigenic preparations. The test is widely used in immunological and other biological research, laboratory diagnosis of diseases, pregnancy tests, and forensic analyses.

Principle

Immunodiffusion test is based on a simple but effective principle that two opposing concentration gradients are formed between the wells by diffusion of antigen and antibody if they were placed side by side in two adjacent wells in a semi solid agar medium. At the point of optimum concentration (Zone of equivalence) of antigen and antibody, a line of precipitation will form within 18–24 hours somewhere between the two wells. Different geometrical patterns between antiserum and antigen wells could be observed depending on the similarity between the tested antigens as illustrated below.

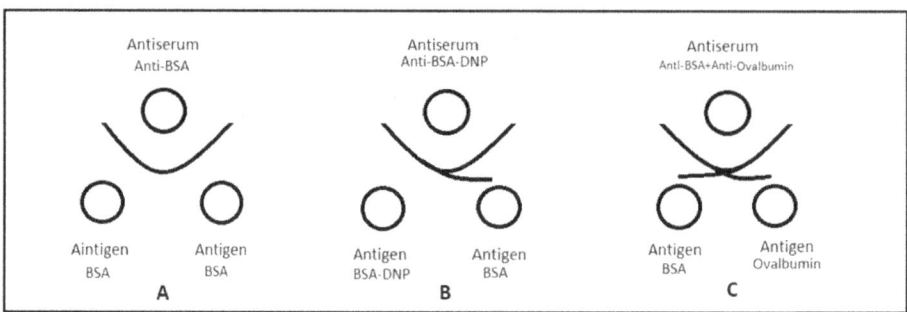

Figure 5.1 Double Immunodiffusion: Patterns of Precipitins

(BSA = Bovine Serum Albumin; BSA-DNP = BSA-2,4 Dinitrophenol(hapten); Ovalbumin = Egg white)

Pattern of Identity: A The antibodies in the antiserum react with both the antigens resulting in a smooth line (line of confluence) of precipitates. The antibodies are specific for the two antigens or in other words the two antigens are immunologically identical. (Fig.5.1: A)

Pattern of Partial Identity: B In the 'pattern of partial identity', the antibodies in the antiserum react more with one of the antigens than the other. The 'spur' is thought to result from the additional antigenic determinant (DNP) present in one antigen (showing 'spur') but lacking in the other antigen. (Fig.5.1: B)

Pattern of Non-Identity: C In the 'pattern of non-identity', One set of antibodies in the antiserum specific to/react with antigenic determinants of one antigen (BSA) and another set of antibodies to that of the other antigen (Ovalbumin) indicating the two antigens are immunologically unrelated/nonidentical. (Fig.5.1: C)

Materials

- Slides
- Petri dishes/glass plates
- Pipettes
- Gel punchers
- Micropipette and tips

- BSA
- 0.5% melted agar
- 1.2 % melted agarose in PBS (pH 7.2)

Procedure

1. Glass slides are pre-coated with agarose.
   (**Pre-coating**: To facilitate good adhesion of the gel to the glass slide it is necessary to first coat the slide with a thin layer of 0.2 - 0.5% agar by adding about 0.5 ml to cover entire surface of slide or by brushing the hot agar solution on to the surface of a slide using a brush or cotton and drying the coated slide in a hot air oven for a minutes. The slide can be dried and stored at room temperature until used).

2. Four ml of molten 1.2 % agarose is poured on to the pre-coated glass slide kept on a **levelled** surface (Air bubbles should be avoided).
3. After agarose solidifies, three pairs of 3mm wells are punctured as shown in figure 5.2
4. Ten μl each of 10-fold diluted protein antigen (e.g. BSA) are added in the three antigen wells.
5. Ten μl each of the antiserum are added into the three antiserum wells.
6. The slide is kept inside a Petri dish, with water soaked cotton and then incubated at 37°C for 24 hours/until the precipitate becomes visible and stationary.
7. Check for white precipitation lines as a sharply defined arc in the contact zone of antigen and antibody.

Note: Interpret the lines with reference to Zone of Equivalence.

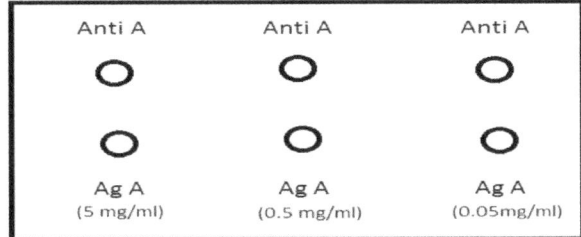

Figure 5.2 Indicative pattern for adding antigen and antibodies for double diffusion.

Exercise: Draw the patterns of precipitin lines you are likely get in the figure given below.

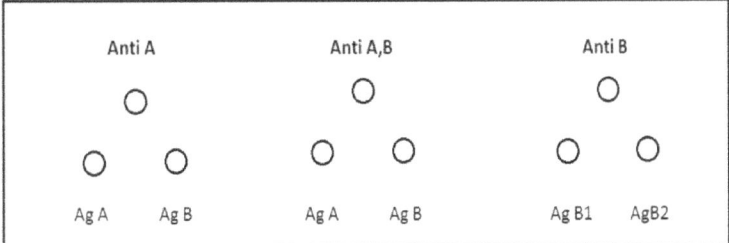

Reference

1. Ouchterlony O. Antigen-antibody reactions in gels. Acta Pathol Microbiol Scand. 1949. 26(4):507-15.

................................Notes/Records ....

5.2 MANCINI SINGLE RADIAL IMMUNODIFFUSION (SRID)

Introduction

Single Radial Immunodiffusion (SRID) is a simple quantitative assay to determine the concentration of an antigen. By using different concentrations of an antigen, a standard curve is obtained from which the unknown amount of an antigen in a sample can be quantified. This test is commonly used in the clinical laboratory for the determination of immunoglobulin levels in patient samples.

Principle

The antibody is incorporated into the agar and antigen is placed in the well cut in the agar. The antigen diffuses outwards and radially, eventually becoming stationary at the zone of equivalence forming a ring of precipitation around the well. Since the diameter of the ring is directly proportional to the concentration of antigen, a standard curve can be constructed to determine unknown concentrations of the same antigen.

Materials

- Glass plates (7 X 10 cm preferred)/ glass slides
- Gel punch
- Petri dish
- Cotton
- Micropipette and tips

- Antigen
- Specific antibody
- 1% melted agarose in PBS (pH 7.2) (see appendix)
- Alcohol (70% ethanol)

Procedure

1. Glass slides are wiped with 70% ethanol to make it grease free and are pre-coated with agarose.
2. 10 ml of 1% agarose in PBS is melted to dissolve completely.
3. The molten agarose is cooled to 55°C.
4. 120µl of antiserum is added to 6ml of agarose and gently mixed for uniform distribution of the antiserum.
5. The agarose-antibody mixture is poured over the glass plate to form a 1.5 mm thick gel layer.
6. 2 mm wells (6 wells) are punctured as shown in the figure 5.3 (at least 10 mm apart) in the gel.
7. 20µl of standard antigen (e.g. BSA 5mg/ml) of 5-fold dilutions added in 1-4 wells.
8. 20 µl of the antigen of unknown concentrations are added to 5 and 6 wells.
9. The slides are kept inside a Petri dish with water soaked cotton and incubated at 4°C for 24 to 72 hours/ until the precipitates become stationary.

10. Circle of precipitin lines can be seen around each of the wells, which corresponds to the concentration of the antigen.

11. Diameter of the circles is measured using magnifying lens and plastic ruler and a standard graph with diameter of precipitin circle as the function of standard antigen concentration is prepared from which the concentration of the unknown concentration of antigen can be calculated.

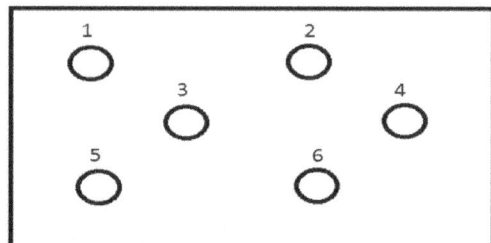

Figure 5.3 Single Radial Immunodiffusion. Indicative pattern for adding standard antigen. Samples 1, 2, 3, 4 – decreasing/increasing concentrations of standard antigen (e.g BSA) to make standard graph. Samples 5, 6 –antigen (e.g BSA) of unknown concentrations.

Reference

1. Mancini G, Carbonara A O & Heremans J F. Immunochemical quantitation of antigens by single radial immunodiffusion. Immunochemistry. 1965. 2:235-54.

·· **Notes/Records** ··

5.3 COUNTER CURRENT IMMUNOELECTROPHORESIS

Introduction

Counter current immunoelectrophoresis is somewhat similar to Ouchterlony double immunodiffusion technique but much faster as it is electrically driven and more sensitive as both the antigen and antibody are oppositely charged and so driven towards each other.

Principle

Counter current immunoelectrophoresis is a rapid qualitative test for the presence of antigen or antibody. The antigen and antibody are (must be) oppositely charged and so when placed appropriately in the gel, on electrophoresis, they move towards each other to meet and form prominent line of precipitation. Since the (biological) reagents are electrically driven the technique is more sensitive and much faster than double immunodiffusion (DID) and is particularly useful for antigens that are in small quantity and that normally diffuse slowly in the gel. The one limitation in this technique is that the test antigen should have anodal mobility (i.e. it should be negative, e.g. BSA) since immunoglobulins (antibodies) have cathodal mobility.

Materials

- Electrophoresis unit with power pack
- Glass slides (7.5 cm X 5 cm)
- Gel punch
- Level table

- 1.5% agarose in PBS (see appendix)
- Phosphate buffered saline (PBS) (see appendix)
- Antigen (e.g. BSA 1mg/ml)
- Antiserum

Procedure

1. Glass slides are pre-coated with agarose.
2. 10ml of 1.5% of agarose is poured on to a glass plate and allowed to solidify for 15min.
3. Four wells of 3mm diameter are punctured on the gel with the gel puncher, as shown in the figure 5.4
4. The slides are placed in the electrophoresis tank and it is filled with electrophoresis buffer till the buffer just touches the gel surface. (The addition of excess buffer should be avoided).
5. 10µl of antigen (e.g. BSA, 1mg/ml) is added in the two wells at the cathode side (negative electrode).
6. 10µl of anti-BSA antiserum (one from immunized rabbit –raise or purchased and the other from control unimmunized rabbit; fish tetramer IgM does not precipitate) are added in the wells at the anode side (positive electrode).

7. The electrophoresis is carried out by connecting the power cord to the electrophoretic power supply (50 V).

8. After 45 mins, the presence and absence of precipitin lines between the antigen and antibody wells are examined and explained.

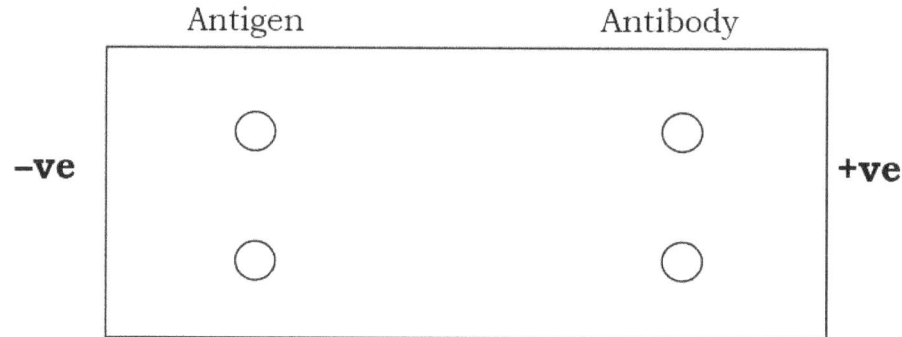

Figure 5.4 Indicative Pattern for addition of antigen and antibody for counter current immunoelectrophoresis.

Reference

1. Ling IT, Cooksley S, Bates PA, Hempelmann E, Wilson RJ. Antibodies to the glutamate dehydrogenase of Plasmodium falciparum. Parasitology. 1986. 92 (Pt 2):313-24.

.... **Notes/Records** ....

5.4 ROCKET IMMUNOELECTROPHORESIS

Introduction

Rocket immunoelectrophoresis is a quantitative method for estimating serum proteins (antigens) and it involves electrophoresis of antigen into a gel containing antibody; the technique is restricted to detection of antigens (that are net negative like BSA) that move to the positive pole on electrophoresis. Low enzyme (protein) concentration can be determined quantitatively using rocket immunoelectrophoresis, and more clearly, if the resolved peaks are transferred electrophoretically to a nitrocellulose membrane and immunostained.

Principle

In rocket immunoelectrophoresis, the antiserum is incorporated into agar and protein antigen is taken in the wells. When an electric current (electrophoresis) is applied, the antigen migrates anodally in the agar. In the beginning, soluble antigen-antibody complexes are formed due to excess of antigen. After some time of migration, the zone of equivalence is reached and an insoluble precipitate is formed which may continue to migrate as more antigen reaches it. An end point is reached when the precipitate can no longer migrate as antigen in the well is exhausted, a phenomenon called 'stable arc' which usually looks like a rocket. The height of the 'rockets' is proportional to the concentration of original antigen sample.

Materials

- Electrophoresis unit with power pack
- Water bath
- Gel punch
- Glass plates (7cmx10cm)
- Leveling table

- 1.5% agarose in PBS (see appendix)
- Antigen (BSA)
- Antiserum (Rabbit anti-BSA antiserum)
- Phosphate buffered saline (PBS) (see appendix)

Procedure

1. Glass plates (7cmx10cm) are pre-coated with agarose.
2. 1ml of antiserum (anti-BSA) is added to 10ml of 1.5% warm (not hot) agarose solution (taken in a 20 ml beaker) ('hand bearable' temperature). It is mixed well for the uniform distribution of antiserum.
3. The mixture is poured onto a glass plate placed on a perfectly even horizontal surface and it is allowed to solidify.
4. 3mm wells (3-4) as shown in figure 5.5 are punctured in the gel with the gel puncture in one edge of the plate.

5. 10µl of antigen (e.g. BSA 1mg/ml with (geometrically or doubly) decreasing concentration (1, 0.5, 0.25 and 0.125mg/ml) are added to the wells (the wells are loaded rapidly to minimize diffusion from the well).

6. The glass plate is placed in the electrophoresis tank. The wells are placed in the cathode (negative electrode) side.

7. The electrophoresis tank is filled with electrophoresis buffer (Phosphate buffered saline) till it touches the gel.

8. Electrophoresis is done at 50 volts, till the rockets are visible or the dye front reaches the edge. This generally takes 60 to 90 minutes.

9. After the rocket is visible, the electrophoresis process is stopped and the glass plates are removed from the electrophoresis tank.

10. The height of the rocket is measured from the upper edge of the well to the tip of the rocket.

11. A standard curve is plotted by taking the height of the rocket on Y-axis (linear scale) against the concentration of antigen on X-axis (log scale) on a semi- log graph sheet or linear scale on a normal graph sheet.

12. The unknown concentration of the antigen in the test sample is determined by the height of the rocket as the function of concentration in the standard curve.

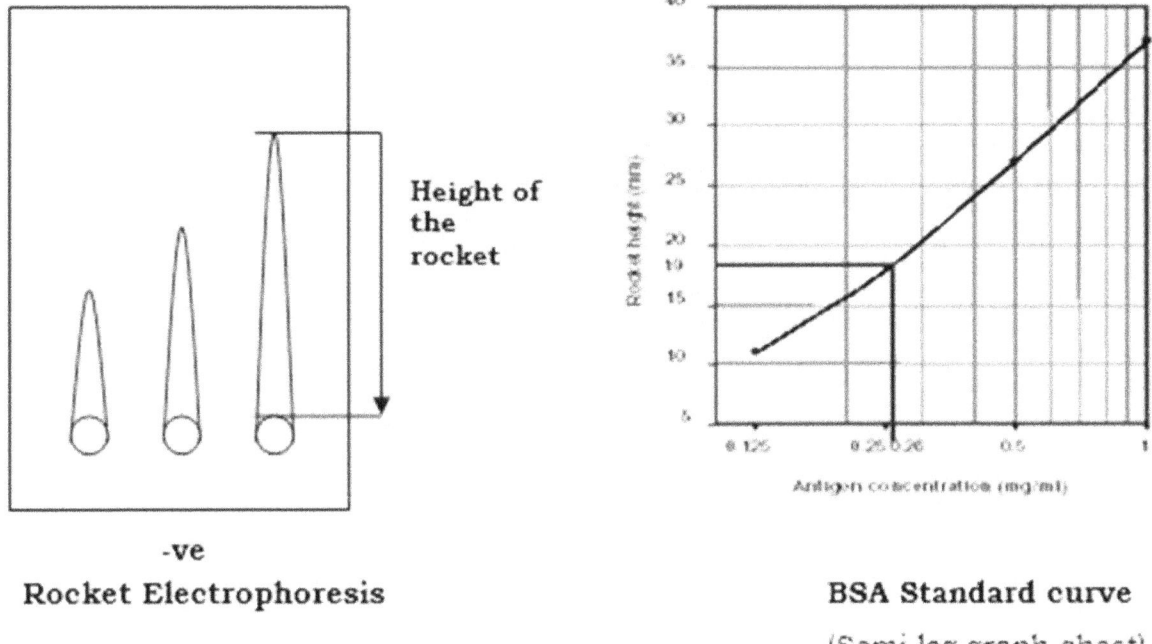

Rocket Electrophoresis

BSA Standard curve

(Semi log graph sheet)

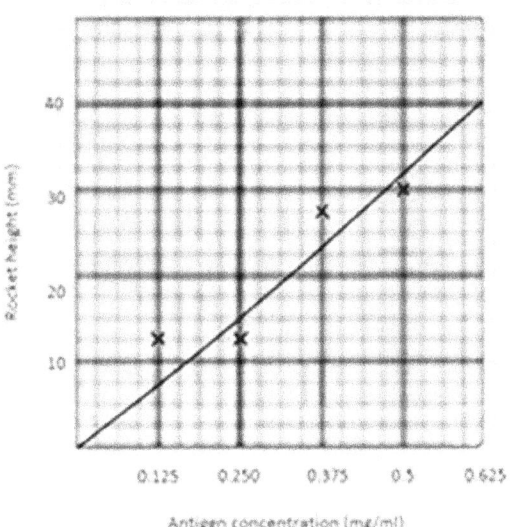

BSA Standard curve

(normal graph sheet)

Figure 5.5 Rocket Immunoelectrophoresis.

Reference

1. Walker JM. Rocket immunoelectrophoresis. Methods Mol Biol. 1984; 1:317-23.

.... **Notes/Records** ....

6. SPECIFIC CELL MEDIATED IMMUNITY (CMI)

As explained in the section 3, the specific (acquired or adaptive) immunity of the vertebrates is divided into humoral immunity which is mediated by substances (antibodies) present in humors of the body (blood and lymph) and Cell mediated immunity mediated by T cells or their cytokines (lymphokines/interleukins). The effector T cells include T_C (T cytototoxicity) and T_{DTH} (T delayed tupe hypersensitivity). Examples of cell mediated immune responses include allograft rejection and delayed type hypersensitivity reaction. In mouse (mammal), these responses can be demonstrated by skin allograft rejection and food pad thickening respectively. In fish, they can be demonstrated by scale allograft rejection and caudal peduncle thickening.

6.1 SCALE ALLOGRAFT REJECTION IN FISH

Introduction

Allograft rejection in vertebrates is considered as an example of cell– mediated immune response, since T- cells (Tc) have the major role in the reaction. In fish, scale allografting and autografting can be performed to demonstrate the rejection of allograft and so the cell mediated immune response.

Principle

The present procedure involves transplantation of scale from one fish to another fish of the same species (allograft) and transplantation of scale from one site to another site of the same fish (autograft). Rejection of the scale in the former (allograft) and acceptance of the scale in the latter (autograft) will demonstrate the allogenic (antigenic) differences between the individuals of an out-bred fish species used. Scale transplantation is performed by inserting scale in the dermal scale pockets after removal of the original scales. Plucking of a scale from its pocket involves the removal of

1. the epidermis covering the exposed portion of the scale plate,
2. the dermis underlying the epidermis and its capillaries, chromatophores etc.,
3. the osteogenic and fibrogenic cells that invest the scale plates and
4. the scale plate and guanophores (reflecting layer) lying beneath it.

Materials

- Fine forceps
- Petri dishes or embryo cups
- Compound microscopes
- Microscopic slides

- Adult fish weighing 25 – 30 g (As per requirement)
- Saline 0.15N
- MS222 or 2-Phenoxyethanol (anaesthetic agent)

Procedure

1. Three or four experimental fishes are placed in a tub/bucket of water with the anaesthetic (MS222) at a concentration of 60mg/lit of water or 2-Phenoxyethanol (100 ppm). The fishes become quiescent in about 20 minutes.

2. A shallow watch glass or Embryo cup with saline is prepared to briefly keep one or two scales to be transplanted.

3. **For autografting,**

   a) Two or three scales from the dorsal pigmented region of the fish are plucked and kept in saline (embryo cup).

   b) Two or three scales (in a row of scales, only alternate scales are removed so that newly grafted scales in that region will be held by the adjacent scales) from the ventral unpigmented region of the same fish are plucked and removed.

   c) One by one, the pigmented scales from the saline are inserted into the empty dermal scale pockets in the ventral region.

4. **For allografting,**

   a) Two or three scales are plucked from the dorsal pigmented region of the donor fish and kept in saline.

   b) From the recipient fish, 2 or 3 scales from the ventral unpigmented region are removed (in row of scales, only alternate scales are to be removed).

   c) One by one the scales from the saline are inserted into the empty dermal scale pockets in the ventral region of the recipient fish.

   d) Rejection (disintegration) or acceptance of scale allograft can be observed 3 days after the transplantation. The grafted scales are observed under binocular/stereo microscope and the changes if any, are noted.

Note: Autograft, being from the same individual, is expected to be accepted and the allograft, being from another individual, to be rejected.

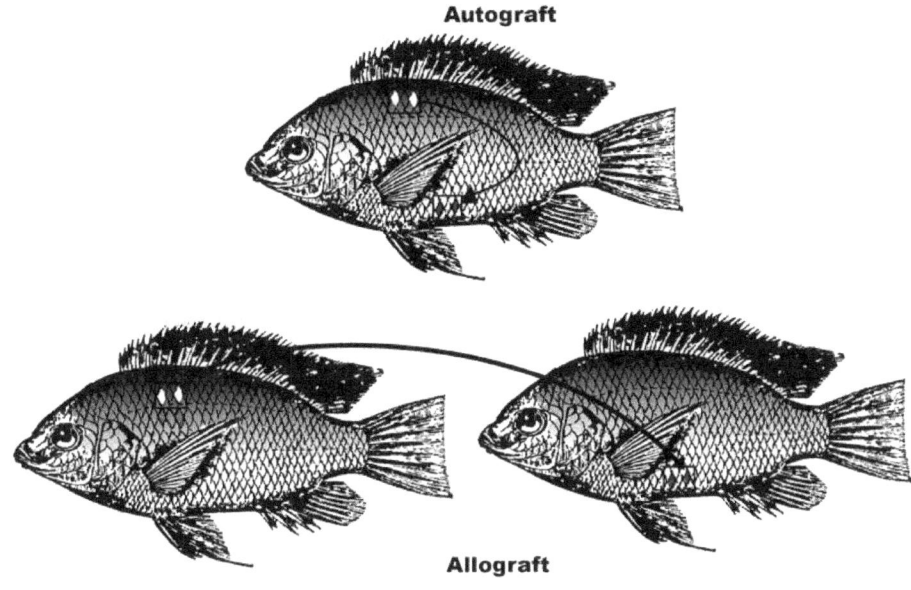

Figure 6.1 Scale grafting in fish.

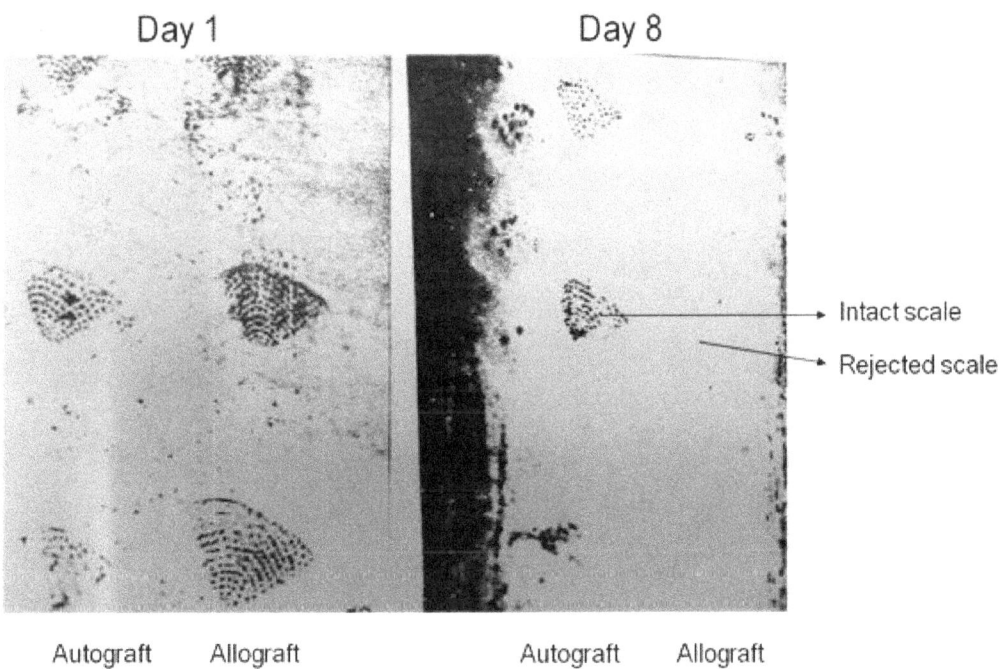

Figure 6.2 Acceptance of autograft and rejection of allograft. Day 1: three autografts (left side) and three allografts (right side) healed after transplantation. Day 8: Accepted autografts with intact melanophores and rejected allografts (Sailendri, 1975).

Reference

1. Sailendri 1975 Ph.D. Thesis submitted to Madurai Kamaraj University, Madurai, India.

.... **Notes/Records** ....

6.2 DEMONSTRATION OF DTH IN FISH (CAUDAL PEDUNCLE THICKENING)

Introduction

Delayed type hypersensitivity (DTH) is called so, because it takes two to three days to develop and it is the only T-cell mediated hypersensitivity (all others are B-cell mediated). DTH was first described by Robert Koch in 1890 upon observing localized inflammatory response developed by tuberculosis patients administered with an intradermal injection of filtrate derived from *Mycobacterium tuberculosis* culture. DTH is very important for protecting host against intracellular pathogens.

Principle

Upon injecting Freund's complete adjuvant (FCA) intraperitoneally in to fish, the peptides from the inactivated intracellular pathogen, *Mycobacterium tuberculosis* (a component of FCA) get associated with MHC-II molecules of APCs (Antigen Presenting Cells) of the fish and are presented to its Th cells. Th1 cells are responsible for DTH. Th1 cells upon sensitization with the antigen, undergo activation and clonal expansion. This process may take approximately 3 weeks in fish (in mammals, 5 days). A booster (FCA) may be given now (around 3 weeks) to elicit higher DTH response later. IFN-γ and IL-2 are the principal cytokines that play a central role in DTH response. When activated Th1 cells encounter the antigen (FCA, now injected into the caudal peduncle) associated with MHCII for the second time via APCs, they secrete several cytokines and chemokines to recruit macrophages to the caudal peduncle resulting in its thickening. The key cytokines secreted include IFN-γ, TNF-β, IL-2, IL-3, and GM-CSF (granulocyte macrophage-colony stimulating factor). Chemokines include IL-8 and MIF (migration inhibitory factor). The recruited macrophages get activated by these cytokines that produce not only surface molecules like MHCII, TNF receptors etc. but also cytotoxic free radicals like reactive oxygen and nitrogen species to destroy the target cells containing *M. tuberculosis*. Since macrophages need to be recruited to the infected site and activated, the hypersensitivity process takes 48-72 hours (hence called DTH).

Materials

- 2 ml syringes with 24G needles
- Vernier calliper

- Tilapia 40-50g (As per requirement)
- Freund's complete adjuvant (FCA) and Freund's incomplete adjuvant (FIA)
- PBS

Procedure

1. Prepare two separate emulsions of FCA and FIA by mixing them separately with PBS in 1:1 ratio (1st emulsion: 1.5 ml FCA +1.5 ml PBS and 2nd emulsion: 1.5 ml FIA +1.5 ml PBS). This can be done either by passing through needleless syringe many times or by vigorous vortexing. The stability/quality of the emulsion prepared can be verified by placing a drop of it in PBS. If the drop does not disperse/ dissolve but floats in PBS, then it indicates emulsion is ready for injection.

2. Group of 10 fish are injected intraperitoneally with 0.2 ml of FCA emulsion per fish. A control- group of 10 fish is injected with 0.2 ml FIA.

3. After 3 weeks, fish were again injected intraperitoneally with FCA and FIA emulsion (0.2 ml per fish) to treated and control- fish respectively (Booster).

4. Two weeks after booster, delayed type hypersensitivity is induced by injecting both the groups with 0.2 ml FCA to the caudal peduncle. This injection is subcutaneous that can be administered just 2-3 mm below the lateral line of the peduncle region of fish.

5. At different time points, (at 0-24-48-72) hours width (in mm) of caudal peduncle are measured and recorded using a Vernier calliper (maximum reaction is expected to occur after 48 hours).

The experimental group injected with FCA is expected to show thickening of caudal peduncle and no thickening is expected in the control group (FIA injected).

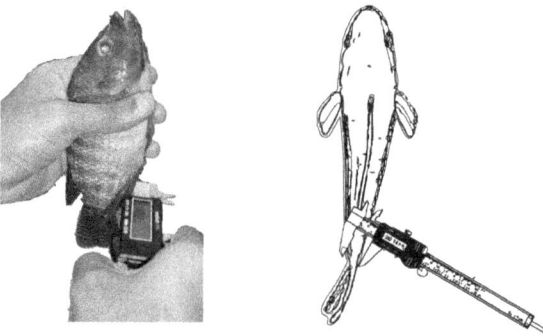

Figure 6.3 Measurement of Caudal Peduncle Thickening using Vernier Calipers.

Note: Why there is no caudal peduncle thickening in FIA injected control ? Write down your response in the 'Notes' space provided below.

Reference

1. Stolen JS. Techniques in Fish Immunology: FITC 1. SOS Publications. 1990.

2. Nakanishi T, Toda H, Shibasaki Y, Somamoto T. Cytotoxic T cells in teleost fish. Dev Comp Immunol. 2011. 35(12):1317-23.

3. Shibasaki Y, Hatanaka C, Matsuura Y, Miyazawa R, Yabu T, Moritomo T, Nakanishi T. Effects of IFNγ administration on allograft rejection in ginbuna crucian carp. Dev Comp Immunol. 2016. 62:108-15.

.... **Notes/Records** ....

7. SEPARATION OF T AND B-LYMPHOCYTES

To study various immune reactions of T and B lymphocytes like antibody or interleukin production, proliferation on treatment with mitogens etc, they have to be first separated from blood or lymphoid organs. In the section 1, the separation of leucocytes (including lymphocytes) from lymphoid organs is explained. Here the separation of lymphocytes from the blood and separation of T and B lymphocytes from the separated lymphocytes are described.

7.1 SEPARATION OF LYMPHOCYTES FROM WHOLE BLOOD

Introduction

As explained above, this is a technique by which lymphocytes can be separated from whole blood drawn/collected from fish . This allows testing of separated lymphocytes for their immune reactions. Further, the isolated lymphocytes can be separated into T lymphocytes and B lymphocytes by other procedures, for further specific studies on the reactions/activities of T and B lymphocytes.

Principle

Heparinized fish blood is diluted 1:1 with blood collection medium (RPMI-1640) so that on centrifugation the blood cells would sediment easily with minimum lymphocyte entrapment. The diluted blood is layered on the lymphocyte separation solution and the preparation is centrifuged to achieve the separation of lymphocyte from the rest of the blood in the form of whitish ring in the inter-phase of diluted plasma and the lymphocyte separation solution. The method of separation is based on the density of the cells separated and called density gradient separation. In fish, this method yields predominantly lymphocytes with > 90% purity.

Materials

- Cell culture medium (RPMI 1640 supplemented with 4mM L-Glutamine, 3% pooled tilapia serum, 100 IU/ml Penicillin and 100 µg/ml Streptomycin)
- Wash medium (RPMI 1640 supplemented with 10 IU/ml Sodium heparin, 100 IU/ml Penicillin and 100 µg/ml Streptomycin.)
- Blood collecting medium (RPMI 1640 supplemented with 50 IU/ml Sodium heparin, 100 IU/ml Penicillin and 100 µg/ml Streptomycin)
- Ficoll gradient (Hisep™, HiMedia, Mumbai, India)
- Sterile centrifuge tubes, needles and syringes
- Ice pack

Procedure

Separation of Peripheral blood lymphocytes

Note: Switch on the cooling centrifuge before going in for bleeding the fish for separation of leucocytes/lymphocytes. All media, chemicals and cells should be maintained at 4°C.

1. Approximately 300 µls (minimum requirement) to 500 µls of peripheral blood are collected from common cardinal vein using 5ml syringe fitted with 24 or 26 gauge needle and pre-filled with 2ml of well mixed blood collecting medium and kept in an ice pack.

2. The needle is removed from the syringe carefully and the diluted blood is carefully laid onto an equal volume (2ml) of Ficoll gradient (Hisep™, HiMedia, Mumbai, India) in a sterile centrifuge tube.

3. The tube is centrifuged at 4°C at 1800rpm for 20mins.

4. After centrifugation, peripheral blood leucocytes in the interface is carefully collected and re-suspended in 2 ml of wash medium in a sterile centrifuge tube.

5. The tube is mildly vortexed and centrifuged at 4°C at 1500rpm for 10mins. The procedure is repeated once again.

6. The cells are then re-suspended in 2ml of cell culture medium and centrifuged at 1500rpm for 10mins at 4°C.

7. The supernatant is removed and the cells are re-suspended in 1ml culture medium and vortexed well.

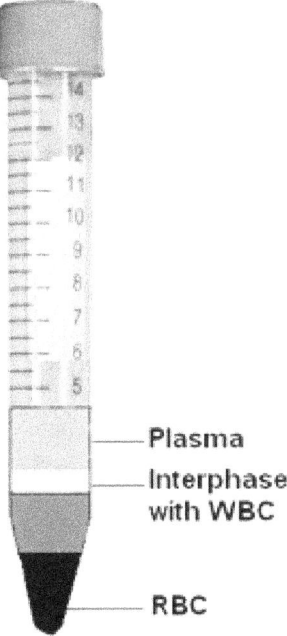

Figure 7.1 Separation of peripheral blood leucocytes from diluted blood using density gradient centrifugation.

References

1. Böyum A. Isolation of mononuclear cells and granulocytes from human blood. Isolation of mononuclear cells by one centrifugation, and of granulocytes by combining centrifugation and sedimentation at 1 g. Scand J Clin Lab Invest Suppl. 1968. 97: 77-89.

2. http://himedialabs.com/TD/LS001.pdf Last retrieved 11-04-2018.

.... **Notes/Records** ....

7.2   NYLON WOOL SEPARATION OF T AND B LYMPHOCYTES

Principle

B cells have surface immunoglobulins (IgM) and other surface markers like CD 19. The B cells become sticky when treated with warm saline (37°C). This property is exploited to separate B cells from T cells. The lymphocytes earlier separated by density gradient centrifugation, are added on to a nylon wool column. When warm saline is added into the nylon wool column, all B cells stick to the nylon wool fibre and all the 'non-sticky' T cells are eluted. Then, cold saline is added into the nylon wool column which results in B cells becoming 'non-sticky' and get eluted.

Materials

- Incubator
- Water bath
- Centrifuge
- Microscope
- Microscopic slides
- Drinking straw
- Nylon wool
- Forceps
- Petri dish
- Micropipette (50 - 500µl)
- Pasteur pipette
- Eppendorf tubes
- Icebox

- Physiological saline (see appendix)
- RPMI – 1640 medium
- Ice

Preparation of Nylon wool column

1. 12 – 14 cm of drinking straw is takcn.
2. On one end of the straw a slanting cut was made and sealed by slightly heating the tip in flame.
3. Nylon wool fibres are finely teased using a pair of forceps and the teased fibres are loosely packed into the straw.
4. The packed nylon wool column is washed by adding 5 ml of physiological saline.
5. A small opening is made at the sealed end of the straw to drain the Physiological saline.
6. After washing with Physiological saline, the nylon wool column is filled with 3 ml of RPMI – 1640 medium in a horizontal position.
7. The nylon wool column is kept in the incubator (at 37°C for 30 minutes) in horizontal position. This process activates the nylon wool column.

Separation Procedure

8. The Ficoll gradient-separated lymphocytes (suspended in medium) are loaded or transferred into the activated nylon wool column.

9. Then the column is held vertically above an Eppendorf tube and warm saline (37° C) is slowly dripped into the column. The warm saline passing out of the column (containing non-sticky T lymphocytes) is collected in an Eppendorf tube.

10. After warm saline elution of T lymphocytes, now cold saline (22° C) is dripped through the column. The column is gently squeezed to release the adhered B cells (the process is repeated twice).

11. The cold saline dripping out of the column containing B lymphocytes is collected in another Eppendorf tube.

Note: The presence or absence of B cells in eluted samples can be confirmed by positive or negative anti-Ig immunoflourescence respectively if the appropriate facilities are available.

References

1. Scharsack JP, Steinhagen D, Kleczka C, Schmidt JO, Körting W, Michael RD, Leibold W, Schuberth HJ. The haemoflagellate *Trypanoplasma borreli* induces the production of nitric oxide, which is associated with modulation of carp (*Cyprinus carpio* L.) leucocyte functions. Fish Shellfish Immunol. 2003 Mar; 14(3):207-22.

2. Scharsack JP, Steinhagen D, Kleczka C, Schmidt JO, Körting W, Michael RD, Leibold W, Schuberth HJ. Head kidney neutrophils of carp (*Cyprinus carpio* L.) are functionally modulated by the haemoflagellate *Trypanoplasma borreli*. Fish Shellfish Immunol. 2003 May; 14(5):389-403.

3. P.C. Blaxhall, The Separation and Cultivation of Fish Lymphocytes, In Fish Immunology, edited by Margaret J. Manning and Mary F. Tatner, Academic Press, 1985, Pages 245-259, ISBN 9780124692305.

4. C. Findlay M. F. Tatner. A comparative study of T and B lymphocytes in rainbow trout (Oncorhynchus mykiss) following their separation by nylon wool adherence and lectin agglutination techniques. Comparative Haematology International. 1994. 4:55-60.

.... **Notes/Records** ....

8. IMMUNOBLOTTING (WESTERN BLOTTING)

Introduction

In Biology, the term "blotting" refers to the transfer of biological samples from a gel to a membrane and their subsequent detection on the surface of the membrane. The western blot was described by W. Neal Burnette, of Fred Hutchinson Cancer Research Centre in Seattle, Washington in 1981. The specificity of the antibody-antigen interaction enables a single protein to be identified amid a complex protein mixture. Western blotting is commonly used to positively identify a specific protein in a complex mixture and to obtain qualitative and semi quantitative data about that protein. This method is, however, dependent on the use of a high-quality antibody directed against a desired protein.

Principle

The basic principle behind Western blotting and immuno-detection is that of antigen and antibody interaction. An antigen bound to the primary antibody is detected by a secondary antibody (specific to primary antibody) labelled with an enzyme which on addition of the (chromogenic) substrate gives a coloured insoluble product, which can be detected visually.

The proteins from bacterial cells, tissue culture, blood or any other source are first separated by SDS-PAGE and are transferred (blotted) from the gel to a nitrocellulose or nylon membrane that binds proteins non-specifically. When this membrane is treated with primary antibody and if the specific antigens are present, then the antibody will bind to them. Then the added enzyme -labelled secondary antibody recognizes and binds to the primary antibody. The antigen-primary antibody-secondary antibody-enzyme complex is detected when the enzyme converts a soluble, colourless substrate into an insoluble, coloured product (Figure 8.1). Thus, the coloured bands appear on the white membrane wherever a protein antigen interacts with the specific primary antibody.

Materials

- Western Blot apparatus and accessories

A. SDS- PAGE

- Acrylamide stock (30%)
- 1.5 M Tris-HCl (pH 8.8)
- 1M Tris-HCl (pH 6.8)
- 10% Ammonium Persulphate
- 10% SDS

- TEMED (N, N, N', N'-Tetramethylethylenediamine)
- Glycine
- Sample Buffer 4X
- Water saturated n-butanol

Note: Polyacrylamide gel is the product of acrylamide and N, N-methylenebisacrylamide polymerization (Bis, for short). Acrylamide is the main ingredient to which Bis is cross-linked to form the gels. After mixing acrylamide and Bis in required proportions, polymerization is initiated by the addition of ammonium per sulphate. DTT or TEMED is added in very small quantity to increase the speed of polymerisation (catalyst). The total amount of acrylamide (%T) and Bis (%C) determines the relative size of the pores formed within the gel. As the amount of monomers (%T and %C) increases, the size of the pores decreases. The size of the pores in turn determines the separation of molecules electrophoresed.

Rule of thumb The smaller the size of the protein of interest, the higher the percentage of polyacrylamide (mono:bisacrylamide) and *vice versa.*

B. WESTERN BLOTTING

- PBS (10X)
- Transfer Buffer
- Blocking solution
- Primary antibody
- Secondary antibody
- Developing solution

I. Preparation of stocks

a. Acrylamide 30% (100 ml)

- Acrylamide : 29.2g
- N-N bis acrylamide : 0.8 g

The above-mentioned substances are dissolved in 100ml sterile distilled water and stored in brown bottle at 4°C.

b. 1.5M Tris-HCl

18.171 g Tris is dissolved in 100 ml water. The pH is adjusted to 8.8 using HCl until it stabilizes. Then it is filtered through Whatman No.1 filter paper and autoclaved. (Note: Tris-HCl can be stored at room temperature).

c. 1M Tris-HCl

6.057g Tris is dissolved in 50 ml water. The pH is adjusted to 6.8 using HCl until it stabilizes and then filtered through Whatman No.1 filter paper and autoclaved. (Note: Tris-HCl can be stored at room temperature)

d. 10% SDS

- 10g SDS is dissolved in 100 ml of distilled water.

e. SDS gel running buffer

- Tris   : 3 g
- Glycine   : 14.4 g
- SDS   : 1 g

The required amounts of Tris and Glycine are dissolved in 200 ml of distilled water. 1 g of SDS is added and allowed to settle and dissolve. Make up to 1000 ml.

f. Sample loading buffer 4X for 5 ml

- 1M Tris HCl (pH 6.8)   : 2.1 ml
- 20% SDS   : 1.0 ml
- 100% Glycerol   : 1.0 ml
- β- Mercapto ethanol   : 0.5 ml
- Bromophenol blue (0.05%)   : 2.5 mg

The above-mentioned substances are dissolved and made up to 5ml with sterile distilled water.

g. Water Saturated Butanol

Equal volume of n-butanol is added to distilled water and mixed well and allowed it to stand for 10 minutes.

h. 10% APS

- 0.1g of ammonium per sulphate is dissolved in 1ml of water.
- Precaution: APS to be freshly prepared before every use

i. 5% Stacking gel (2ml)

- 30% Acrylamide   : 0.33 ml
- 1.0 M Tris (pH- 6.8)   : 0.25 ml
- 10% SDS   : 0.02 ml
- 10% APS   : 0.02 ml
- TEMED   : 0.002 ml

The above-mentioned substances are dissolved and made up to 2ml with sterile distilled water.

j. 10% Separating gel (5ml)

- Acrylamide   : 1.7 ml
- 1.5MTris (pH-8.8)   : 1.3 ml
- SDS   : 0.05 ml
- APS   : 0.05 ml
- TEMED   : 0.002 ml

The above-mentioned substances are dissolved and made up to 5ml with sterile distilled water.

k. 10X PBS (1 L)

- NaCl : 80g
- KCl : 2g
- Na_2HPO_4 : 11.5g
- KH_2PO_4 : 2g
- Distilled water : 1000ml

l. Transfer Buffer (1 L)

- 25mM Tris : 2.9g
- 190mM Glycine : 14.5g
- 20% Methanol : 200ml
- Dissolved in 1X PBS. : 800ml

m. Blocking Solution

- 5% non-fat dry milk and 0.1% Tween 20 are dissolved in 1x PBS

n. Staining solution

- Coomassie Brilliant Blue (R-250) : 0.001 %
- Methanol : 50 %
- Acetic acid : 7 %

o. Destaining Solution

- Methanol : 50 %
- Acetic acid : 7 %

Procedure

A. Separation of proteins using SDS-PAGE

1. All reagents except ammonium per sulphate (APS) and TEMED were taken in a container to prepare **separating gel monomer solution**. The container is gently swirled to deaerate solution after adding each reagent in order to remove oxygen which interferes with polymerisation.

2. Add APS and TEMED and mix well by swirling gently just before pouring the monomer solution into the assembled glass plates up to 3/4ᵗʰ of the plate height.

3. After adding separating gel solution, immediately overlay it with 1 ml of water without mixing with the gel by a steady, even rate of delivery.

4. Polymerization of gel takes about 45 minutes to 1 hour. After polymerization, water overlaying the gel was drained with strips of filter paper.

5. **Stacking gel** monomer solution is prepared similar to that of separating gel.

6. Pour the solution up to the top of the plate and promptly place a comb on top of it. 8. Allow the gel to polymerize for 15 minutes and remove the comb.

9. Finally, the gel assembly is placed in the buffer chamber and running gel buffer is added into the chamber.

10. Prepare the samples by boiling at 100°C with an equal volume of sample buffer for 3-5 mins. Electrophoresis is done at 80-100 V till the dye front reached the bottom of the gel.

11. After electrophoresis, gel is kept in the staining solution (0.001 %-Coomassie brilliant blue R-250) for 2 h or overnight and the excess stain is removed by destaining till the bands were clear.

B. Transferring Proteins From the Gel to Nitrocellulose Membrane (Fig. 2)

1. Cut about six numbers of Whatman no.1 filter papers to be used as absorbent and the nitrocellulose membrane should be cut to the exact size of the gel.

2. Soak the membrane and filter papers in the transfer buffer before stacking for transfer.

3. On a solid plastic platform, stack two pieces of wet absorbent paper. Place another absorbent paper on the gel in the plate and slowly transfer the gel on to the stack, placing the gel side up.

4. Place the wet nitrocellulose membrane on the gel, aligning the edges and keep the remaining absorbent paper on the stack. (Gel and membrane are sandwiched between stacks of filter paper).

5. Remove all the air bubbles between the layers by rolling a pipette from the centre to the edges.

6. Position the transfer sandwich to the electro blotter in such a way that the membrane is near the positive electrode. Screw the plates of the apparatus.

7. Pour the transfer buffer into the transfer apparatus and connect the electrodes and set the power supply to ~ 60mA. Transfer is done for one hour.

Note: More transfer tips:

1. The gel needs to equilibrate for 15-30 minutes in transfer buffer. Failure to do so will cause shrinking while transferring, and a distorted pattern of transfer.

2. Membranes should not be touched with bare hands as oils and proteins present in fingers may block transfer and/or create dirty blots. Plastic tweezers can be used instead.

3. After sandwiching the gel and membrane between paper, carefully remove air bubbles between the gel and membrane by rolling them out with a pipette or 15 ml tube. Alternatively, assembling the sandwich in a dish of transfer prevents air bubble formation.

4. Buffer is added to prevent formation of bubbles in the first place. Wear gloves!

5. Membrane and filter papers used during transfer must be of same size as that of the polyacrylamide gel. Large overhangs may interfere with current passing through the membrane in semi dry transfers.

C. Immunological Detection of Protein

1. After transfer, the membrane is washed with blocking solution (5% milk powder in 1XPBS) for twenty minutes. Discard the solution and this washing is repeated for 2-4 times.

Note: Membranes used in blotting experiments have a high capacity to bind proteins. Hence it is necessary to block the membrane to prevent the primary and/or secondary antibodies from non-specifically binding to the membrane.

2. Then dilute primary antibody (1:500) in 30 ml of blocking solution. Rock the membrane and primary antibody mixture gently for 45 min- 1hr.

3. After incubation, discard the solution and the membrane is washed with 1XPBS for three times.

4. Then dilute secondary antibody (Alkaline phosphatase conjugated goat anti-rabbit antibodies) as (1:1000) in 30 ml of the blocking solution. Rock the membrane and secondary antibody mixture gently for 1hr.

5. After incubation, discard the solution and the membrane is washed with 1X PBS for three times.

6. Develop the membrane in dark by adding about 20 ml of developing solution (BCIP/ NBT solution- Generally, BCIP/NBT Phosphatase Substrate deposits a permanent, dark purple stain on membrane sites bearing phosphatase)

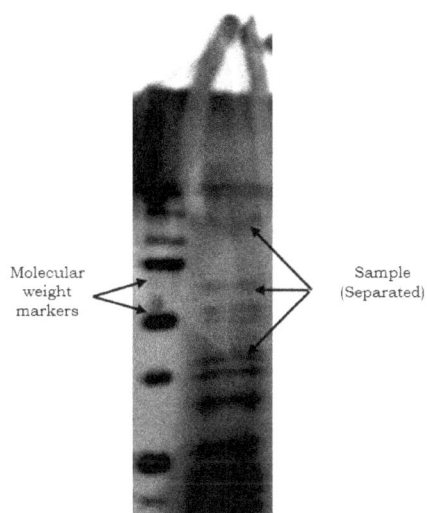

Figure 8.1 Separation of proteins using SDS-PAGE

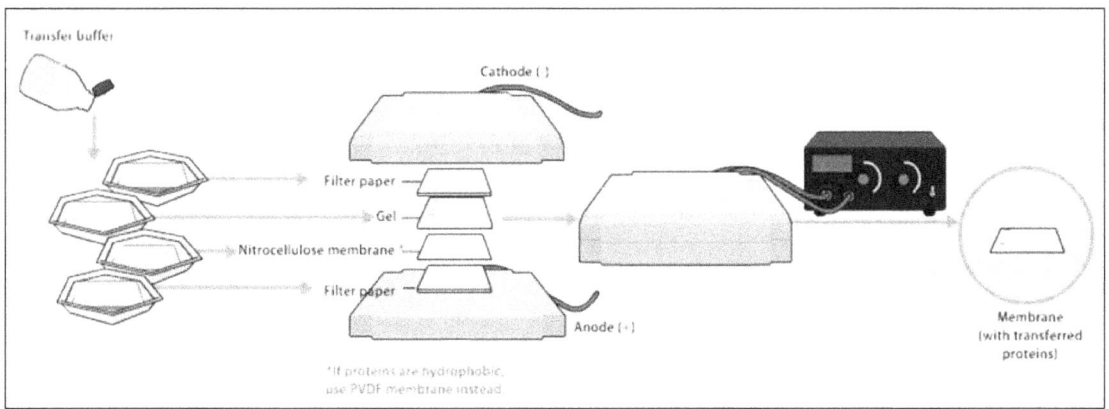

Figure 8.2 Transferring proteins from the gel to nitrocellulose membrane (courtesy, Bensaccount at English Wikipedia [CC BY 3.0 http://creativecommons.org/licenses/by/3.0)], via Wikimedia Commons)

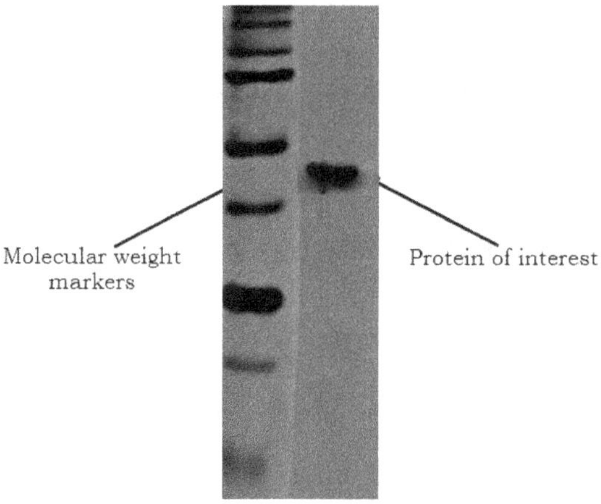

Figure 8.3 Immunological detection of protein (using labelled specific antibody)

Reference

1. Kurien BT, Scofield RH. Western blotting. Methods. 2006 Apr;38(4):283-93.
2. Kurien BT, Scofield RH. Western blotting: an introduction. Methods Mol Biol. 2015; 1312:17-30.

.... **Notes/Records** ....

9. GENE EXPRESSION ANALYSIS OF IMMUNE RELATED GENES

Gene expression is a fundamental process by which different proteins such as enzymes, cytokines, surface receptors and signaling molecules were produced. Expression of immune related genes is modulated by many factors like infection, vaccination and immunostimulation. An immunostimulant modulates the immune system by altering the gene expression pattern of immune related genes like various interleukins, interferons etc. Modulation of gene expression is both dose and time dependent process. RT-PCR is a sensitive method to quantify the degree of modulation in gene expression brought about by an immunostimulant.

Macromolecular immunostimulants like polysaccharides and polynucleotides are recognized by pattern recognition receptors like TLRs (Toll like receptors or TLRs are protein receptors present on immune cells like macrophages and dendritic cells) which in turn modulate the expression of immune related genes by activating transcription factors like NF-κB. On the other hand, small molecules like curcumin etc. can directly activate NF-κB resulting in modulation of gene expression. Analysis of gene expression is a sophisticated technique which gives a number of information on cellular, tissue function and even host-pathogen interaction.

9.1 RNA ISOLATION AND CDNA SYNTHESIS

Introduction

The first step in gene expression analysis is the isolation of total RNA from the cell/ tissue in its purest form possible. The quality of RNA used generally decides the outcome of the analysis. This isolation can be done by various methods of which the 'Trizol™' is widely followed. Trizol™ is a commercially available phenol, chloroform mixture that requires no prior processing of cells/tissues. The method is rapid and takes only 20-25 minutes. It is a simple phase separation method in which hydrophilic RNA remain in the upper aqueous phase while hydrophobic macromolecules such as DNA, proteins etc. remain in the lower phenol: chloroform phase. The upper layer is removed carefully with a pipette and extracted with suitable chemicals to isolate pure RNA.

Principle

Semi-quantitative Reverse Transcriptase PCR (RT-PCR) is a rapid and inexpensive technique to quantify gene expression at mRNA level. In this method, total RNA of a cell/ tissue/organ (transcriptome) is isolated that includes mRNA, rRNA, tRNA etc. Of the total RNA content, mRNA is specifically converted to cDNA using oligo dT primers and reverse transcriptase enzyme. This is because only mRNA possesses a polyA tail. The converted cDNA is then amplified using gene specific primers in a PCR. The amplified products are then size separated in agarose gels and visualized using fluorescent dyes such as Ethidium bromide (EtBr). The intensity of EtBr increases with the amount of DNA that can be densitometrically quantified using ImageJ software.

Materials

- Spectrophotometer with 260 and 280 nm wavelength filters
- Teflon micro-pestles
- 1.5 ml centrifuge tubes, 0.2 ml thin walled PCR tubes
- Sterile forceps
- Refrigerated centrifuge
- Mini centrifuge (spinwin)
- Thermal cycler
- Horizontal electrophoresis unit
- Gel doc system with software
- Personal computer with ImageJ software
- Centrifuge stands for 1.5 ml and 0.2 ml
- Ice bucket
- Mini cooler -20 °C
- Reagent bottles and measuring cylinders
- Tissue paper, gloves and trays
- Micropipette (1, 200, 50, 10 µl volumes)

- Organs isolated from control (PBS) and MacroGard (MG) treated fish
- Trizol
- Chloroform
- Isopropanol
- Ethanol
- Distilled water
- cDNA synthesis kit
- Red dye PCR master mix
- Agarose
- 50X Tris Acetate buffer
- Ethidium bromide

Procedure

RNA isolation

1. Equal amount (weight) of experimental (treated) and control tissue samples are taken in 1.5 ml centrifuge tubes.
2. Trizol (typically 1 ml or just to submerge the organ) is added to the tube.
3. Homogenize with Teflon micro-pestle until the organ now looks like a cell suspension.
4. Keep the suspension at room temperature for 5 min to facilitate complete lysis of cells.

5. After 5 min, 0.2 ml chloroform per ml Trizol (added initially) is added and vortexed vigorously till a precipitate of milky white consistency is reached.

6. Incubate the Trizol-chloroform mixture for 2 min at room temperature.

7. After incubation, centrifuge at 12,000 xg for 10 min at 4 °C.

8. Carefully transfer the clear, upper aqueous layer into a fresh 1.5 ml centrifuge tube and keep it in ice bucket. Discard the remainder layers and pellet.

9. To the separated aqueous layer, 0.5 ml isopropanol is added per ml of Trizol (added initially).

10. Incubate on ice for 1 min to facilitate precipitation of RNA from the aqueous layer.

11. Centrifuge the tubes at 12,000 xg for 10 min at 4 °C.

12. Discard the supernatant and the pellet is washed with 1 ml of ethanol per ml of Trizol.

13. Ethanol is then separated by centrifuging at 7,500 xg for 10 min at 4 °C and discarding the supernatant.

14. The pellet contains RNA which is then dissolved in double distilled water by heating it at 55 °C.

15. Dissolved RNA is quickly checked for quality in spectrophotometer by taking 260/280 nm ratio. If the ratio is >1.9, it indicates 100% purity. Typically, a ratio of at least 1.5 to 1.6 is expected to conduct reverse transcription.

cDNA synthesis

1. For cDNA synthesis, the following reaction mixture is prepared (according to Qiagen, Valencia, USA). This recipe may change between manufacturers and it is advised to follow the manufacturer's instructions (given below).

Reagent	Volume
10X RT buffer	2 µl
dNTP mix	2 µl
oligo dT primer (10 µM) (must be obtained separately)	2 µl
Reverse transcriptase	1 µl
RNA template	1 µl
Double distilled water	12 µl
Total	**20 µl**

2. The reaction mixture is then incubated at 37 °C for 1 hour to synthesize cDNA.

PCR

1. For PCR amplification of immune related genes, it is advisable to use gene specific primer sequences available in the literature. If that information is not available, one should design one's own primers and validate it by sequencing the amplified products.

2. For PCR amplification, the following reaction mixture is prepared (according to Sigma). This recipe may change between manufacturers and it is advised to strictly follow the manufacturer's instructions (given below)

Reagent	Volume
Red dye master mix	10 µl
Forward primer (1 µM)	1 µl
Reverse primer (1 µM)	1 µl
cDNA	1 µl
Water	7 µl
Total	**20 µl**

Agarose gel electrophoresis

1. A 50X TAE buffer solution can be prepared by dissolving 242g Tris base in water, adding 57.1mL glacial acetic acid, and 100mL of 500mM EDTA (pH 8.0) solution, and bringing the final volume up to 1 litre with double distilled water.
2. Dilute 50X TAE buffer to 1X by adding 10 ml of it to 490 ml of double distilled water.
3. Prepare 2% agarose by adding 2 g of agarose in 100 ml 1X TAE buffer.
4. Dissolve agarose by heating to boil in a microwave oven.
5. Let the agarose solution cool and in the mean-time seal the gel electrophoresis boat with cellophane tape.
6. After agarose cooled to a palm bearable temperature 10 µl of 10 mg/ml ethidium bromide solution is added.
    Caution: Ethidium bromide is a known carcinogen.
7. Immediately pour the agarose solution containing ethidium bromide into the sealed boat and place appropriate gel comb immediately.
8. Leave the set up away from light for 15-20 min to allow complete solidification of the agarose gel.
9. After solidification, the gel boat is placed inside the electrophoretic chamber and filled with 1X TAE. Enough TAE is added to submerge the gel completely.
10. PCR amplified products were then loaded into the gel using a micropipette.
    Note: Be careful to add equal volumes of all products into the respective wells.
11. Electrophoresis is then carried out by passing appropriate (50-100 V) voltage to the electrophoresis apparatus till the dye front reaches the bottom of the boat.
12. Electrophoresed gels are then carefully placed on the stage of a transilluminator or gel doc instrument and photographed with the help of a digital camera/smartphone or gel doc software respectively.

.... **Notes/Records** ....

9.2   QUANTIFICATION OF GENE EXPRESSION USING IMAGEJ

Introduction

PCR products run in a gel can be quantified after photographing using ImageJ software. ImageJ developed by National Institutes of Health, USA as a pixel statistics software. ImageJ can read a number of picture formats including jpg and tiff and the number of pixels occupied by each band is used to calculate the integrated density values. Integrated density value is an indirect measure of quantity of PCR products which infers the amount of gene expression modulation brought about by control/treatment

Principle

Digital photographs are made up of pixels or small addressable points. When agarose gels containing PCR products are photographed, each band contains a distinct set of pixels that can be quantified using specialized software such as ImageJ. Accurate measurements can be made by drawing a rectangle around the band of interest and then calculating the integrated density value.

Procedure

1. Download ImageJ for Windows from the following link https://imagej.nih.gov/ij/download.html.

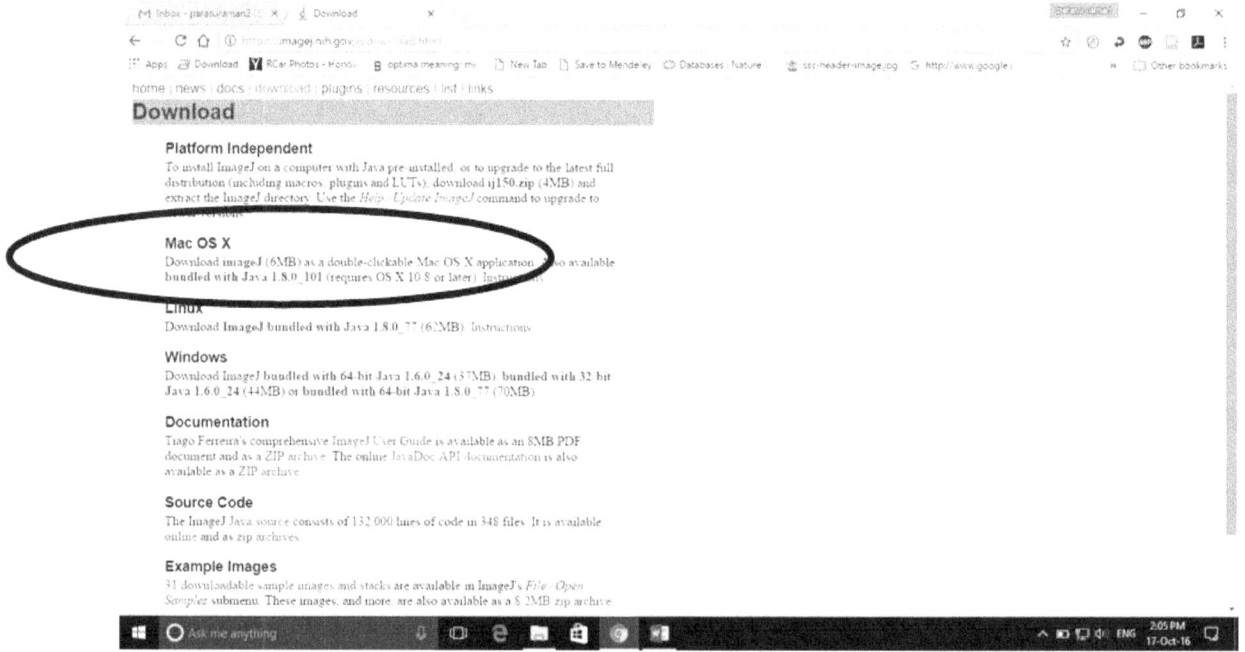

Figure 9.1   Screenshot of webpage for downloading ImageJ software.

2. Open the picture obtained from gel doc clicking File menu and then open (or press ctrl + O from keyboard).

3. Go to Analyse menu and set measurements tool. This will open the following window

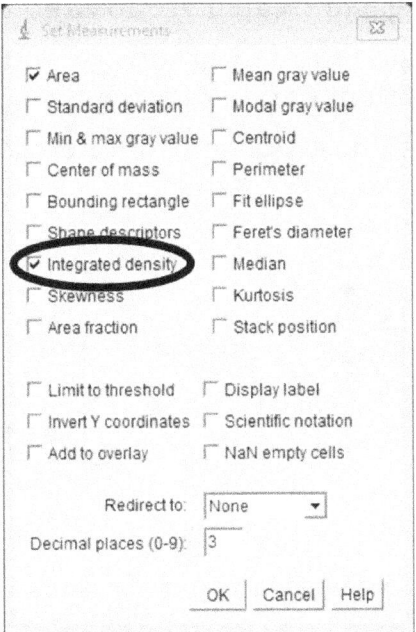

Tick integrated density option.

Figure 9.2 Dialogue box for selecting integrated density in ImageJ

4. Draw a rectangle on the control band first.

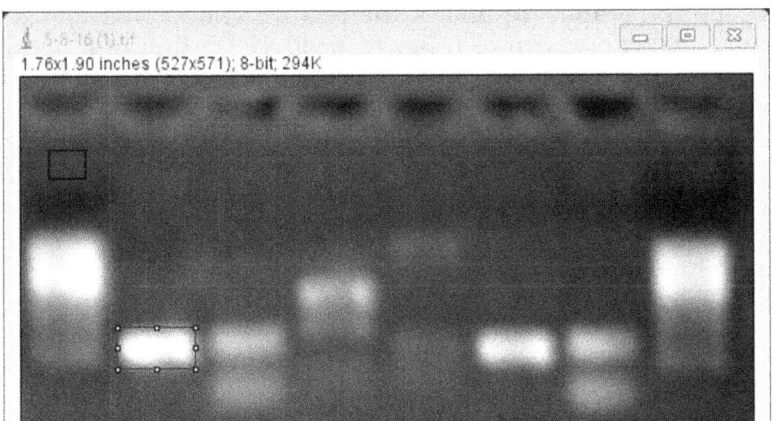

Figure 9.3 Screenshot of drawing a rectangle around band of interest.

5. Then click ctrl + M. This will open a new window that shows "IntDen" value.

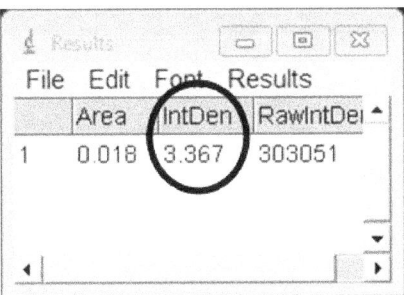

Figure 9.4 Result window containing integrated density values.

6. Drag the same rectangle to treated groups and again press ctrl + M.

7. After measuring all the required groups, results table can be exported from File menu of measurements and choosing Save As option.

8. Finally draw a graph of ratios of gene of interests to the control β-actin band.

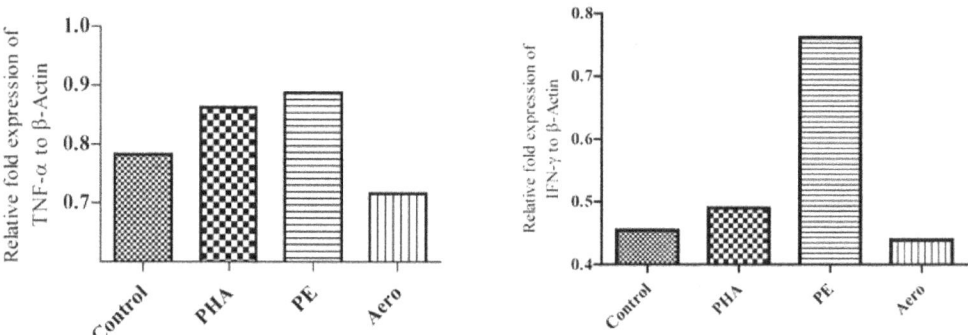

Figure 9.5   Sample gene expression analysis by reverse transcriptase (RT)-PCR. Cells were seeded at an initial concentration of 10^6 cells/well in 6-well tissue culture plates and were left untreated (control) or treated with commercial PHA or *Dendrophthoe falcata* aqueous extract (1:10 dilution in TBS). One hour after treatment, plates were washed twice with ice-cold PBS and cells in each well were lysed with Trizol. The lysate thus obtained was used for RNA preparation and subsequent RT-PCR. Amplified products obtained from RT-PCR were electrophoresed in agarose gels stained with ethidium bromide and photographed using gel doc **(A)**. ImageJ was then used to measure the integrated density and plotting the graph. **(B)** shows the relative fold expression of TNF-α and **(C)** shows the relative fold expression of IFN-γ respectively to that of β-actin. The experiment was repeated three times with leukocytes of different fishes but similar results were obtained.

······························· **Notes/Records** ·······························

9.3   PRIMER DESIGNING

Introduction

Success of PCR experiments depends upon the characteristics of primers such as GC content, annealing temperature, primer melting point etc. In earlier days, all these characteristics were calculated manually which is very cumbersome. Nowadays, software like Pimer3plus can automatically calculate these vital statistics and gives a plenty of primer options from which suitable primers can be selected.

Principle

Primer3 software is a useful, free to use and it is an online interface. Primer3 allows you to screen candidate oligonucleotide against a mispriming Library. Primer3 has many C++ libraries that calculate melting temperature, propensity to form hairpins etc. The user has to give input in boulder IO (text file) and get the primer sequences as output. All the calculations were done online by global Primer3 servers.

Procedure

1. Retrieve a query DNA sequence from the database or user library.
2. Paste the sequence in the sequence box in the Raw format.
3. Choose Task option "Detection".
4. Enter the regions of Excluded regions, Targets and Included region.
5. Click "Pick primer" button.

Result

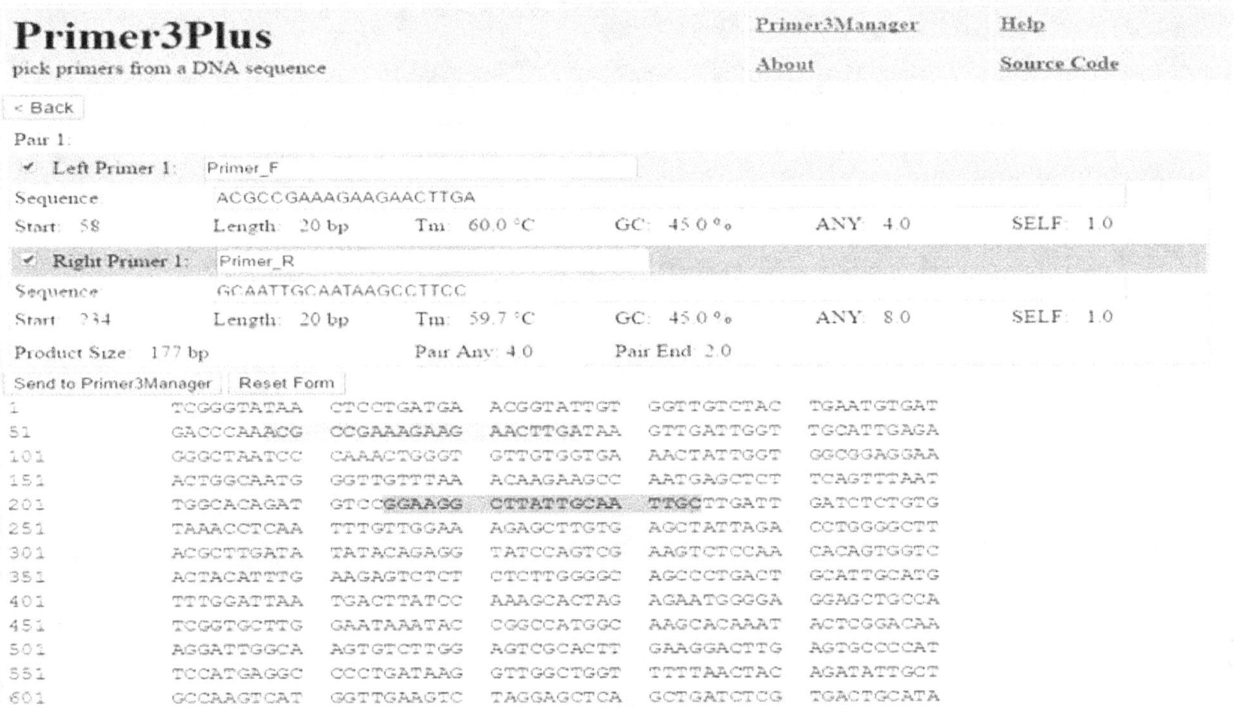

Figure 9.6   Output window showing predicted primers for the given DNA sequence.

Reference

1. Subramani PA, Narasimha RV, Balasubramanian R, Narala VR, Ganesh MR, Michael RD. Cytotoxic effects of Aeromonas hydrophila culture supernatant on peripheral blood leukocytes of Nile tilapia (Oreochromis niloticus): Possible presence of a secreted cytotoxic lectin. Fish Shellfish Immunol. 2016 Nov; 58:604-611. doi: 10.1016/j.fsi.2016.09.061.

.... **Notes/Records** ....

10. NON-SPECIFIC HUMORAL IMMUNE RESPONSES

As in mammals, the immune responses of fishes are of two types, specific immune responses and non-specific immune responses. But being primitive among the vertebrates, fishes, unlike mammals, depend more on non-specific immune mechanisms than specific immunity to protect themselves from infectious pathogens. In fishes, the non-specific immune responses are of two types, humoral responses and cellular responses. Non-specific humoral immune responses include responses mediated by substances present in the humor (fluid) in the body, that is blood (e.g. lysozyme, myeloperoxidase etc) which protect the fish from diseases by reacting with the pathogens that enter the fish . The non-specific cellular immune responses include responses mediated by cells (macrophages and neutrophils etc.) such as phagocytosis, reactive oxygen production(ROS) etc. In this section (10), laboratory exercises for non-specific humoral immune responses are described and in the next section (11) that of non-specific cellular mechanism are dealt with.

10.1   SERUM MYELOPEROXIDASE ACTIVITY

Introduction

Myeloperoxidase (MPO) is a peroxidase enzyme (EC 1.11.1.7) most abundantly present in neutrophils. It is a lysosomal protein stored in azurophilic granules of neutrophil. MPO has a haem pigment, which causes its green colour in secretions rich in neutrophils, such as pus from an infected tissue. In humans, MPO is a 150 kDa protein dimer consisting of two 15 kDa light chains and two variable-weight glycosylated heavy chains bound to a prosthetic haem group. Three isoforms have been identified, differing only in the size of the heavy chains. Upon contact with a pathogen, neutrophils produce a respiratory burst characterized by intense uptake of oxygen. The resulting superoxide dismutates into hydrogen peroxide (H_2O_2). The toxicity of H_2O_2 is greatly enhanced by the haem enzyme myeloperoxidase, which uses H_2O_2 to convert chloride (Cl_2) into hypochlorous acid (HOCl).

$$Cl^- + H_2O_2 + H^+ \rightarrow HOCl + H_2O$$

Remarkably, myeloperoxidase is the only enzyme known to oxidize Cl_2 to HOCl at plasma concentrations of halide. Some reactions of hypochlorous acid lead to further reactive oxygen species with high potential for tissue damage. Hypochlorous acid reacts with hydrogen peroxide to form singlet oxygen and other products (shown below). Hypochlorous acid also reacts with nitrite to yield the powerful chlorinating and nitrating compound, NO_2Cl.

$$+ H_2O_2 \longrightarrow {}^1O_2 + H_2O + H^+ + Cl^-$$

$$+ O_2^- \longrightarrow {}^\cdot OH + O_2 + Cl^-$$

$$HOCl \quad + Fe^{2+} \longrightarrow {}^\cdot OH + Fe^{3+} + Cl^-$$

$$+ NO_2^- \longrightarrow NO_2Cl + {}^-OH$$

Furthermore, it oxidizes tyrosine to tyrosyl radical using hydrogen peroxide as oxidizing agent. Hypochlorous acid and tyrosyl radical are cytotoxic, so they are used by the neutrophil to kill bacteria and other pathogens.

Principle

Serum Myeloperoxidase activity in fish is measured by the method of Quade and Roth (1997) with partial modification (Sahoo *et al.*, 2005). The azurophilic granules in cytoplasm of fish neutrophils contain the enzyme myeloperoxidase (MPO). The enzyme myeloperoxidase that is released from azurophilic granules during the oxidative burst activity is measured through the peroxidase content of the serum or the cells. TMB (3, 3', 5, 5', -tetramethyl benzidine hydrochloride) is oxidized during the enzymatic peroxidase activity. The oxidized product of TMB has a deep blue colour. A clear yellow colour is formed after addition of the acidic stop solution. For detection of oxidized TMB, the OD of the yellow colour is measured in a standard microplate reader at 450 nm after the reaction has been stopped with acid.

Materials

- Microplate reader
- 96-well 'U' bottom microtitre plate

- Sample Serum
- Phenol red-free Hank's balanced salt solution (HBSS) containing Mg^{2+} and EGTA (Ethylene glycol tetra acetic acid)
- TMB (3, 3', 5, 5', -tetramethyl benzidine hydrochloride) - H_2O_2 (Genei, India)
- 2M H_2SO_4

Procedure

1. To 10µl of serum, 90µl of HBBS is added in a 96-well 'U' bottom microtitre plate.
2. To this mixture, 50µl of TMB is added and incubated for 2 minutes at room temperature.
3. To stop the reaction, 50µl of 2M H_2SO_4 is added.
4. Finally, OD is read in a microplate reader at 450nm against 100µl of HBSS as blank.

References

1. Quade, M.J. and J.A. Roth, A rapid, direct assay to measure degranulation of bovine neutrophil primary granules. Vet Immunol Immunopathol, 1997. 58(3-4): p. 239-48.

2. Sahoo, P.K., J. Kumari, and B.K. Mishra, Non-specific immune responses in juveniles of Indian major carps. Journal of Applied Ichthyology, 2005. 21(2): p. 151-155.

.... **Notes/Records** ....

10.2   SERUM LYSOZYME ACTIVITY

Introduction

Lysozyme (muramidase, EC 3.2.1.17) is an important mucolytic enzyme found in many of the leucocytes. Lysozyme is reported from various organisms ranging from bacteriophages, microbes, plants, invertebrates to vertebrates (Jolles & Jolles, 1984). Lysozyme is also found in animal secretions like mucus and saliva, and in the cell vacuoles of plants. Lysozyme causes bacteriolysis by hydrolysing the β (1-4) linkages between *N*-acetylmuramic acid and N-acetylglucosamine in the cell walls (peptidoglycan layers) of Gram-positive bacteria. Lysozyme can also lyse Gram-negative bacteria after their outer cell wall is disrupted to expose the inner peptidoglycan layer by serum complement and/or other enzymes. Apart from the bacteriolytic activity, lysozyme is also shown to promote phagocytosis by directly activating neutrophils and macrophages or indirectly by an opsonic effect. Neutrophils of fish contain large quantity of lysozyme followed by monocytes and macrophages where lysozyme is found in lesser quantity. It is reported that among the organs and tissues, kidneys have highest lysozyme levels, followed in descending order by the alimentary tract, spleen, skin mucus, serum, gills, liver and muscle. Lysozyme is a single polypeptide chain containing about 120 amino acids. Lysozyme of freshwater fish shows a pH optimum of 5.4.

Principle

Lysozyme splits the β (1-4) linkages between *N*-acetylmuramic acid and N-acetylglucosamine in the cell walls (peptidoglycan layers) of Gram-positive bacteria leading to bacteriolysis. Serum lysozyme activity is determined by using the turbidimetric assay described by Parry *et al.* (1965) with the microplate adaptation of Hutchinson and Manning (1996). The assay is based on lysis of lysozyme-sensitive gram positive bacterium, *Micrococcus lysodeiticus*. The extent of lysis is measured by reduction in optical density. One unit of lysozyme activity is defined as a reduction in absorbance of 0.001 per minute (min⁻¹)

Materials

- Centrifuge
- Microplate reader
- Pipette man (Multichannel) – (range 50 - 300μl)
- 96 well Microtitre plate
- Tuberculin syringe (fitted with 24 gauge needle)
- Serological tubes
- Eppendorf tubes

- Fish serum
- *Micrococcus lysodeiticus* (0.3mg ml⁻¹, substrate)
- Phosphate buffered saline (PBS)
- 0.05M sodium phosphate buffer (pH 6.2)

Procedure

1. Samples of blood is taken from the experimental fish (or any animal) with a Tuberculin syringe

2. The blood is collected in serological tubes, stored overnight at 4°C and centrifuged at 1500rpm (600g) for 15 min to separate serum.

3. Separated serum is stored in Eppendorf tubes at minus 20°C until used.

4. Ten microlitres of serum are added to 250µl of the bacterial suspension (*Micrococcus lysoleiticus*) in 96-well microtitre plate.

5. The reduction in absorbance at 490nm is determined after 0.5 and 4.5min of incubation at 28°C in a microplate reader.

6. One unit of lysozyme activity is defined as a reduction in absorbance of 0.001 min^{-1}

Calculation

Difference in OD is for 10µl of serum, for 4 minutes. Hence, calculate for 1 ml of serum and for 1 minute.

$$\frac{\text{Difference in OD} \times 1000 \times 1}{10 \times 4} \text{ (or simply) Difference in OD} \times 25 \text{ units / ml}$$

Precaution   Care should be taken to prevent any bubble formation while adding both the serum and the substrate.

Note: Serum lysozyme activity can also be expressed in micrograms using hen egg white lysozyme as standard.

References

1. Jollès P, Jollès J. What's new in lysozyme research? Always a model system, today as yesterday. Mol Cell Biochem. 1984. 63(2): p.165-89.

2. Parry RM Jr, Chandan RC, Shahani KM. A Rapid and Sensitive Assay of Muramidase. Proc Soc Exp Biol Med. 1965. 119:384-6.

3. Hutchinson, T.H. and M.J. Manning, Seasonal trends in serum lysozyme activity and total protein concentration in dab (*Limanda limanda* L.) sampled from Lyme Bay, U.K. Fish Shellfish Immunol, 1996. 6(7): p. 473-482.

4. Stolen, J.S., Techniques in Fish Immunology: FITC 11990: Sos Publications.

.... **Notes/Records** ....

10.3 ANTIPROTEASE ASSAY

Introduction

Antiproteases are one of the components of non-specific immunity of the vertebrates. Several pathogens invade the host and obtain their nutrients by using their extracellular proteolytic enzymes. To counter/resist this attack, the host tissue and serum contains a range of inhibitors (antiproteases) neutralize the proteolytic enzymes produced by the pathogens. Fish plasma contains several protease inhibitors like α1-antiprotease, α2 antiplasmin and α2 macroglobulin which play an important role in restricting the ability of bacteria to invade the host and grow *in vivo*. Inhibition of trypsin activity is a convenient way of measuring anti-protease activity of the serum.

Principle

The assay uses an aniline - arginine dye ester (BAPNA) as a substrate for trypsin which hydrolyses the aniline dye resulting in a colour change that can be measured photometrically. This chromogenic substrate, Nα-<u>b</u>enzoyl-DL-<u>a</u>rginine-<u>p</u>-<u>n</u>itro<u>a</u>nilide hydrochloride HCl (BAPNA) is hydrolysed by trypsin amidase yielding the yellow dye, paranitroaniline which can be measured photometrically. Protease inhibitors in the sample serum inhibit/reduce the trypsin activity which can be expressed in terms of % inhibition by the serum

Materials

- Microplate reader (Bio-Rad, USA)
- Eppendorf tubes
- Fish serum

- 0.01M Tris (hydroxy methyl) amino methane hydrochloride (Tris HCl)
- 2mM Nα-benzoyl-DL-arginine-p-nitroanilide HCl, (BAPNA, HiMedia)
- Trypsin (Trypsin Bovine Pancreas, in 0.01 M Tris HCl, pH 8.2, Himedia)
- 30% acetic acid

Procedure

1. To 10µl of serum, 20µl of trypsin (1mg/ml in 0.01M Tris HCl) is added in an Eppendorf tube (A2).
2. The above said mixture without serum is maintained as trypsin blank (A1) and Tris HCl without trypsin is maintained as serum blank. Usually serum blank is just used to compare whether colour change occurs or not.
3. The tubes are incubated for 5 min at room temperature
4. To this, 500µl of 2mM BAPNA is added
5. The volume is made up to 1 ml using 0.1M Tris HCl
6. The Eppendorf tubes are incubated for 25 min at room temperature
7. To this mixture, 150µl of 30% acetic acid is added to stop the reaction
8. After that, 300µl of the mixture is taken to read the OD at 410 nm and the OD readings are used in the formula given below to express the results in terms of % Trypsin inhibition.

Calculation

$$\% \text{ Trypsin Inhibition} = \frac{\text{Trypsin blank OD } (A1) - \text{Sample OD } (A2)}{\text{Trypsinblank OD } (A1)} \times 100$$

References

1. Bowden TJ, Butler R, Bricknell IR, Ellis AE. Serum trypsin-inhibitory activity in five species of farmed fish. Fish & Shellfish Immunology 1997 7(6): 377-385.

2. Zuo, X. and Woo, P.T.K. 1997. In vivo neutralization of *Cryptobia salmositica* metalloprotease by alpha 2-macroglobulin in the blood of rainbow trout *Oncorhynchus mykiss* and in brook charr Salvelinus fontinalis. Dis. Aquat. Org. 29, 67-72.

.... **Notes/Records** ....

10.4   SERUM BACTERICIDAL ASSAY

Introduction

Serum bactericidal assay is a rapid, simple and sensitive colorimetric assay developed to evaluate the bacterial killing activity of fish serum against *Aeromonas hydrophila*. The procedure involves the use of the tetrazolium compound, 3-[4, 5-dimethylthiazol-2-yl]-2, 5-diphenyltetrazolium bromide (MTT) which is converted to an insoluble purple formazan by cleavage of the tetrazolium ring by the mitochondrial "Succinate tetrazolium reductase" system

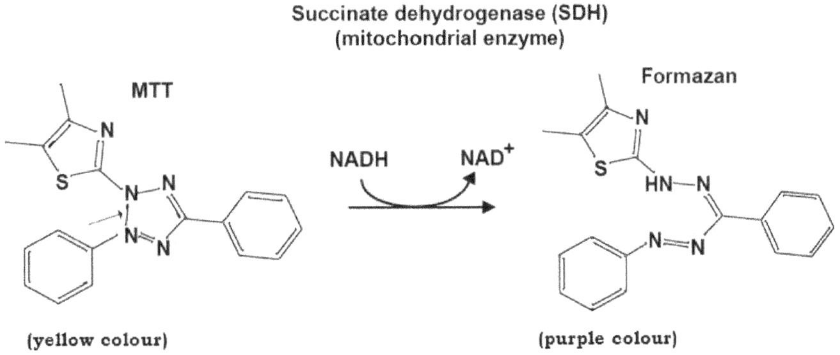

Figure 10.1   Reduction of MTT to formazan by Succinate dehydrogenase

Principle

MTT is reduced to purple formazan precipitate by live *A. hydrophila*. Succinate-dehydrogenase is a mitochondrial enzyme present in the bacteria which reduces the tetrazolium salt MTT into formazan (Welker *et al.*, 2007). Dead bacteria do not react with MTT.

Materials

- 96-well 'U' bottom microtitre plate
- Micropipette
- Microtips
- Centrifuge
- Microplate reader

- Fish serum

- 24hrs *Aeromonas hydrophila* culture
- MTT [3-[4, 5-dimethylthiazol-2-yl]-2, 5-diphenyltetrazolium bromide] solution (2.5 mg/ml)
- Hank's Balanced Salt Solution (HBSS)
- DMSO (Dimethylsulphoxide)

Procedure

1. Twenty microlitres of serum and HBSS (without serum) are taken separately in duplicate wells in a 'U' bottom 96 well microtitre plate.

2. To each of these 4 wells, 20 µl of 24 hrs old *Aeromonas hydrophila* culture is added.

3. Then the titre plate is incubated for 2.5 h at room temperature.

4. Then 25 µl of MTT solution is added to each of these mixtures and incubated for 10 min to allow the formation of formazan precipitate.

5. The plates are centrifuged at 1500 rpm for 10 min and the supernatant is discarded.

6. 200 µl of DMSO is added per well to dissolve the precipitate

7. Purple colour is formed and its intensity is measured colorimetrically at 560nm with a reference filter of 650nm.

8. Results could be interpreted either as absorbance unit or as % control

Note:

Absorbance unit = HBSS Blank O.D – Sample O.D value.

Subtract the absorbance of samples from HBSS control and report as absorbance units corresponding to the bactericidal activity of the serum sample. These absorbance units are proportional to the degree of bactericidal activity.

$$\text{Percent control} = \frac{\text{Sample O.D} \times 100}{\text{Blank O.D}}$$

Reference

1. Welker, T.L., Lim, C., Yildirim-Akosy, M and Klesius, P.H. (2007). Growth, immune function and disease and stress resistance of juvenile Nile tilapia (*Oreochromis niloticus*) fed graded levels of bovine lactoferrin. Aquaculture 262, 156-162.

.... **Notes/Records** ....

10.5   ALTERNATE COMPLEMENT ASSAY

Introduction

Complement is a group of serum proteins that play a vital role in host defence against infections. The complement system is composed of 2 pathways, classical pathway (mediated by specific antibodies) and alternate pathway (ACP) without the involvement of specific antibodies. Thus, for activation of ACP, formation of immune complex or presence of antibody is not required. The alternate complement activity is very high in fish serum compared with that of mammals suggesting this pathway is very important in the defence mechanism of fish.

Principle

The activity of complement in serum sample can be assayed by determining the amount of serum required to lyse erythrocytes provided.

Materials

- Microplate reader (Bio-Rad, USA)
- Cooling centrifuge
- 96-well "U" bottom microtitre plate
- Micropipette and microtips

- Test serum
- Phenol red free Hank's balanced salt solution (HBSS) containing Mg^{2+} and EGTA (see appendix)
- 3 % Sheep Red Blood Cells (SRBC)

Method

1. One hundred microlitres of serum sample is serially double diluted up to 11th well with equal volume of HBSS in a 96 well "U" bottom microtitre plate. Serum samples are added in the row A, B etc up to F (and diluted as mentioned above).
2. To this, 100 μl of 3% SRBC in HBSS is added to all the wells.
3. In rows G and H, 100 μl distilled water (positive control) and 100 μl of HBSS (negative control) were added to 3% SRBC (already added in step 2 respectively. This is done to determine the OD of 100% and 0% haemolysis.
4. The plate is incubated for 1 hour at 22°C.
5. After incubation, the plate is centrifuged at 1500 rpm for 5 min at 4°C.
6. Transfer 200μl of supernatant to fresh plate and the haemoglobin content of the supernatant is assessed by measuring the OD at 540nm.
7. The highest (double) dilution of serum that shows OD slightly higher than that of HBSS is taken as the $\log_2$ titre of alternate haemolytic complement present in the serum and it can be plotted like the way usually done for plotting $\log_2$ antibody titre. The assay can be carried out using serum obtained from minimum three individual fishes and the mean ± SE of $\log_2$ titre can be plotted.

References

1. J. Ortuno, M.A. Esteban, V. Mulero, J. Meseguer. Methods for studying the haemolytic, chemoattractant and opsonic activities of seabream (Sparus aurata L.) serum. A.C. Barnes, G.A. Davidson, M.P. Hiney, D. McIntosh (Eds.), Methodology in fish disease research (1998), pp. 97-100. Aberdeen

2. Alexander CP, Kirubakaran CJ, Michael RD. Water soluble fraction of *Tinospora cordifolia* leaves enhanced the non-specific immune mechanisms and disease resistance in *Oreochromis mossambicus.* Fish Shellfish Immunol. 2010 Nov; 29(5):765-72. doi: 10.1016/j.fsi.2010.07.003.

3. Christybapita D, Divyagnaneswari M, Michael RD. Oral administration of Eclipta alba leaf aqueous extract enhances the non-specific immune responses and disease resistance of Oreochromis mossambicus. Fish Shellfish Immunol. 2007 Oct; 23(4):840-52.

4. Steinhagen D, Helmus T, Maurer S, Michael RD, Leibold W, Scharsack JP, Skouras A, Schuberth HJ. Effect of hexavalent carcinogenic chromium on carp Cyprinus carpio immune cells. Dis Aqua Organ. 2004 Nov 23; 62(1-2):155-61.

5. Prabakaran M, Binuramesh C, Steinhagen D, Michael RD. Immune response and disease resistance of Oreochromis mossambicus to Aeromonas hydrophila after exposure to hexavalent chromium. Dis Aqua Organ. 2006 Mar 2; 68(3):189-96.

.... **Notes/Records** ....

11. NON-SPECIFIC CELLULAR IMMUNE RESPONSES

As explained in the last section, the non-specific immune cellular immune responses are mediated by leucocytes like macrophages and neutrophils. The cellular responses described in this section include production of reactive oxygen species (ROS), reactive nitrogen intermediates and myeloperoxidases by peripheral blood leucocytes like neutrophils and macrophages.

11.1 MEASUREMENT OF INTRACELLULAR REACTIVE OXYGEN SPECIES (ROS) PRODUCTION BY LEUCOCYTES FROM PERIPHERAL BLOOD

Introduction

Cells use multiple cytotoxic systems of which the NADPH oxidase system is a very important component. This enzymatic system consists of several components which, once assembled in the plasma membrane in response to a stimulus, trigger the so-called respiratory burst, in which there is a huge increase in oxygen consumption and the production of large amounts of superoxide anions in neutrophils and other phagocytic cells. Reactive oxygen species (ROS) is a collective term that includes a large variety of free oxygen radicals (e.g. superoxide anion, and hydroxyl radicals) but also derivatives of oxygen that do not contain unpaired electrons (e.g., hydrogen peroxide, hypochlorous acid, peroxynitrite, and ozone). NADPH oxidase system can be activated by phagocytosis and with the aid of other cytotoxic mechanisms. After receptor activation in neutrophils/macrophages, molecular oxygen undergoes a one or two-electron reduction to form superoxide anion (O_2^-) or hydrogen peroxide (H_2O_2). The electron donor, NADPH, is formed by the oxidation of glucose in the hexose monophosphate shunt.

Principle

Neutrophils and macrophages are capable of producing superoxide anions (O_2^-) by the action of NADPH oxidase during respiratory burst activity. The intracellular superoxide anion produced by the cells reduces the Nitroblue tetrazolium salt into an insoluble purple coloured compound, formazan. The formazan can be solubilized using Potassium hydroxide and Dimethyl sulphoxide to give a blue green coloured solution. The colour formed can be read at 655 nm in microplate reader.

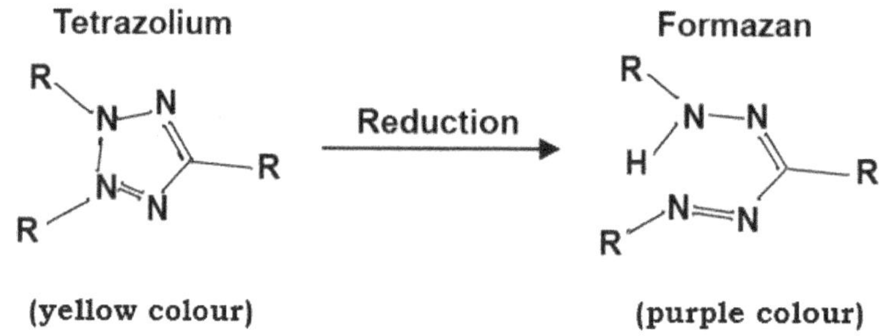

Figure 11.1   Reduction of a tetrazolium to a formazan. The "Rs" stand-in for various organic groups that define the various tetrazolium salts and provide their unique chemical characteristics:

Materials

- Microplate reader
- 96 well flat bottom plates
- Neubauer chamber
- Compound microscope

- Cell culture medium (RPMI 1640 supplemented with 4mM L-Glutamine, 3% pooled tilapia serum, 100 IU/ml Penicillin and 100 µg/ml Streptomycin),

- Wash medium (RPMI 1640 supplemented with 10 IU/ml Sodium heparin, 100 IU/ml Penicillin and 100 µg/ml Streptomycin.)

- Blood collecting medium (RPMI 1640 supplemented with 50 IU/ml Sodium heparin, 100 IU/ml Penicillin and 100 µg/ml Streptomycin.)

- Ficoll gradient (Hisep™, HiMedia, Mumbai, India)
- Trypan blue stain-0.5%in PBS (filter sterilized)
- Nitroblue tetrazolium chloride (NBT) (35mg in 5 ml culture medium)
- Methanol
- Dimethyl Sulphoxide (DMSO)
- Potassium hydroxide
- Phorbol myristate aceate (PMA) (0.14µg/ml) [optional]

Procedure

Separation of Peripheral Blood Leukocytes

Note: Remember to switch on the cooling centrifuge about 30 minutes before going in for dissection or bleeding. All media, chemicals and cells should be maintained at 4°C.

1. Approximately 300 µl (minimum requirement) of peripheral blood is collected from the common cardinal vein using 2ml syringe pre-filled with 1ml of blood collecting medium, mixed well and kept in an ice pack.

2. The needle is removed from the syringe carefully and the diluted blood is carefully laid onto the equal volume of Ficoll gradient (Hisep™, HiMedia, Mumbai, India) in a sterile centrifuge tube.

3. The tube is centrifuged at 4°C at 1800rpm for 20mins.

4. After centrifugation, peripheral blood leucocytes in the interface is collected and resuspended in 2 ml of wash medium in a sterile centrifuge.

5. The tube is mildly vortexed and centrifuged at 4°C at 1500rpm for 10mins. The procedure is repeated once again.

6. The cells are then resuspended in 2ml of culture medium and centrifuged at 1500rpm for 10mins at 4°C.

7. The supernatant is removed and the cells are resuspended in 1ml culture media and vortexed well

8. The cells are incubated at 4°C for 20mins (Time taken for counting cells would also be sufficient).

9. After incubation, the contents are mixed well using a vortexer and 50 µl of cell suspension is mixed with equal volume of trypan blue stain in a sterile Eppendorf tube.

10. The peripheral blood leukocyte suspension is adjusted to contain 40×10^6 cells/ml.

11. Twenty-five microlitre of cell suspension is added to each well in a 96 well flat bottom microplate.

12. Then 25 µl of NBT solution is added (35mg in 5ml culture medium and filtered).

13. The total medium per well is adjusted to contain 175 µl using culture medium (125 µl is added).

14. The microplate is covered with a sterile microplate cover.

15. The plate is incubated in a moist chamber moistened with 1% copper sulphate solution for 2 hrs at 28°C in dark.

16. After incubation, the supernatant is removed and 200 µl of 100% methanol is added for fixing the cells and it is left for 5mins.

17. After incubation 100% methanol is removed and washed with 70% methanol thrice.

18. After washing, the plates are kept for overnight drying.

19. After drying, 125 µl of 2N Potassium hydroxide (KOH) and 150µl of Dimethyl sulphoxide (DMSO) are added per well for dissolving formazan precipitate.

20. Finally, the contents are mixed well to dissolve the precipitate and read the plate at 655nm.

Note:

1. While removing supernatant and washing the microplate, care is taken not to disturb the precipitate in the well.

2. While incubating the microplate, make sure that it is placed well balanced on a flat surface.

3. For finding the effect of PMA on the ROS production, 25 µl of PMA (0.14 µg/ml dissolved in ethanol) is added and consequently reduce the culture medium by 25 µl.

References

1. Secombes CJ. Isolation of salmonid macrophages and analysis of their killing activity. In 'Techniques in fish Immunology.'(Eds J. S. Stolen, T. C. Fletcher, D.

P. Anderson, B. S. Robertsen and W. B. van Muiswinkel). SOS Publications: New Jersey. 1990. pp. 137-154.

2. Steinhagen D, Helmus T, Maurer S, Michael RD, Leibold W, Scharsack JP, Skouras A, Schuberth HJ. Effect of hexavalent carcinogenic chromium on carp *Cyprinus carpio* immune cells. Dis Aqua Organ. 2004 Nov 23; 62(1-2):155-61.

3. Prabakaran M, Binuramesh C, Steinhagen D, Michael RD. Immune response and disease resistance of *Oreochromis mossambicus* to *Aeromonas hydrophila* after exposure to hexavalent chromium. Dis Aqua Organ. 2006 Mar 2; 68(3):189-96.

.... **Notes/Records** ....

11.2 MEASUREMENT OF REACTIVE NITROGEN SPECIES (RNS) BY PERIPHERAL BLOOD LEUCOCYTES

Introduction

The enzyme system responsible for producing Nitric oxide (NO), is Nitric oxide synthase, which exists in three distinct isoforms: i) constitutive neuronal NOS (NOS I or nNOS); ii) inducible NOS (NOS II or iNOS); and iii) constitutive endothelial NOS (NOS III or eNOS which are products of distinct genes located on different human chromosomes (12th, 17th, and 7th chromosomes respectively in humans). Functionally, NOS exists in constitutive (cNOS) and inducible (iNOS) forms. Upon appropriate stimulation, phagocytic cells can form high amounts of nitric oxide (NO) via an increased expression of iNOS. Upon reacting with other superoxides (O_2^-) NO forms peroxynitrite $(ONOO^-)$ which is a potent oxidant. Peroxynitrite in turn produces nitrotyrosine residues. However, tyrosine nitration may also be found after exposure of proteins to nitrite (NO_2^-) in association with hypochlorous acid (HOCl) and myeloperoxidase (MPO) or eosinophil peroxidase (EPO).

Principle

Phagocytic leucocytes produce Nitric Oxide (NO) by the action of inducible nitric oxide synthase enzyme (iNOS). The nitric oxide produced by the cells in cultures is rapidly transformed to more stable nitrite (NO_2^-). The nitrite present in the culture supernatants can be measured colorimetrically by converting it into a pink dye by adding "Griess reagent". Hence it is an indirect measurement of NO production. The culture supernatant must be measured immediately or stored at –20°C, as nitrite formed will be easily oxidized to nitrate.

Intensity of pink dye can be measured photometrically at 570nm. For a reference, a calibration solution with sodium nitrite must be prepared. The calibration (standard) curve has a linear ascent from 0 to 100 µM of nitrite.

Materials

- Microplate reader
- 96 well flat bottom plates
- Cell culture medium (RPMI 1640 supplemented with 4mM L-Glutamine, 3% pooled tilapia serum, 10 IU/ml Penicillin and 100 µg/ml Streptomycin)
- Wash medium (RPMI 1640 supplemented with 10 IU/ml Sodium heparin, 100 IU/ml Penicillin and 100 µg/ml Streptomycin.)
- Blood collecting medium (RPMI 1640 supplemented with 50 IU/ml Sodium heparin, 100 IU/ml Penicillin and 100 µg/ml Streptomycin.)
- Sodium nitrite
- Sulphanilamide
- Naphthyl ethylene diamine dihydrochloride
- Phosphoric Acid (85%)

Preparation of standard curve

Dissolve 69mg of sodium nitrite in 100ml of distilled water (0.01M). From this solution, 100 µl is mixed with 9.9ml (9900 µl) of culture medium to make a stock solution (0.0001M or 100µM). Using this stock solution, a standard curve is generated as described in the table below.

Table 11.1 Preparation of nitrite standards

Culture medium	Nitrite Stock solution (100µM)	Nitrite Concentration
1000µl	0µl	0µM
950µl	50µl	5µM
900µl	100µl	10µM
750µl	250µl	25µM
500µl	500µl	50µM
250µl	750µl	75µM
0µl	1000µl	100µM

Composition of Griess reagent

- Sulphanilamide -1% (w/v)
- Naphthyl ethylene diamine dihydrochloride -0.1 %(w/v)
- Phosphoric acid -2.5 %(v/v)
- Dissolve the above substances in distilled water

Procedure

The whole procedure of plating the cells should be carried out in an aseptic condition. Hence absolute care is needed.

1. The peripheral blood leukocyte suspension (as described earlier) is adjusted to contain 40×10^6 cells/ml (1 million cells in 25 µl per well).
2. 25 µl of cell suspension is added to each well in a 96 well flat bottom microplate.
3. The total medium per well is adjusted to contain 175 µl-using culture media (150 µl medium is added)
4. The microplate is covered with a sterile microplate cover.
5. The plates are incubated in a moist chamber moistened with 1% copper sulphate solution for 4 days at 28°C.
6. After incubation 50 µl of culture supernatant aseptically transferred onto a separate microplate without disturbing the cells underneath.
7. To the culture supernatant equal volume of Griess reagent (50 µl) is added and the plate is left for 10 mins at room temperature for colour development.

8. Pink colour is formed in the culture supernatant and its intensity is measured colorimetrically at 570nm with a reference filter of 650nm.

9. The microplate containing the culture supernatant should be measured immediately or should be stored at -20°C.

Note:

1. While incubating the microplate, make sure that it is placed at well-balanced flat surface.

2. The colour formed is stable for 1 hr only.

3. The Griess reagent and Sodium nitrite solution cannot be stored for more than one day at 4°C.

4. Every time a separate standard graph should be prepared using sodium nitrite since the colour formed varies according to the batch of culture medium used.

References

1. Green LC, Wagner DA, Glogowoski J, Skipper PL, Wishnok JS, Tannenbaum SR. Analysis of nitrate, nitrite and [15N] nitrate in biological fluids.Analytical Biochemistry 1982; 126: 131-138.

2. Alexander CP, Kirubakaran CJ, Michael RD. Water soluble fraction of *Tinospora cordifolia* leaves enhanced the non-specific immune mechanisms and disease resistance in *Oreochromis mossambicus*. Fish Shellfish Immunol. 2010 Nov; 29(5):765-72. doi: 10.1016/j.fsi.2010.07.003.

3. Christybapita D, Divyagnaneswari M, Michael RD. Oral administration of Eclipta alba leaf aqueous extract enhances the non-specific immune responses and disease resistance of Oreochromis mossambicus. Fish Shellfish Immunol. 2007 Oct; 23(4):840-52.

.... **Notes/Records** ....

11.3 MEASUREMENT OF INTRACELLULAR MYELOPEROXIDASE (MPO) ACTIVITY OF LEUCOCYTES FROM PERIPHERAL BLOOD

Introduction

The neutrophils can be distinguished from other leucocytes by the presence of myeloperoxidase (MPO) in their cytoplasmic granules. MPO catalyses the oxidation of halide ions by H_2O_2 to form hypohalites, chloramines and singlet oxygen. Such highly reactive oxygen products have been implicated as microbicidal agents within the phagocytes, either by themselves or in concert with lysosomal enzymes.

$$Cl- + H_2O_2- + H+ \xrightarrow[MPO]{} HOCl + H_2O$$

Principle

The assay is a direct, rapid and quantitative method to assess the degranulation process in neutrophils. The assay is based on MPO- H_2O_2 oxidation of 3, 3', 5, 5'-tetramethylbenzidine (TMB) (Palic *et al.*, 2005). TMB when oxidized becomes blue coloured. The reaction can be stopped using acid solution resulting in a yellow coloured solution. Both the coloured solutions can be measured colorimetrically. If kinetics of the reaction is of your interest, the blue coloured solution can be measured at 655 nm in different time points within a few minutes before the solution reaches the upper detection limit. Otherwise, more commonly, the reaction is stopped 2 min after adding TMB and the yellow coloured solution is measured at 450 nm.

Materials

- Elisa plate reader
- 96 well flat bottom plates

- Cell culture medium (RPMI 1640 supplemented with 4mM L-Glutamine, 3% pooled tilapia serum, 100 IU/ml Penicillin and 100 µg/ml Streptomycin)

- Wash medium (RPMI 1640 supplemented with 10 IU/ml Sodium heparin, 100 IU/ml Penicillin and 100 µg/ml Streptomycin)

- Blood collecting medium (RPMI 1640 supplemented with 50 IU/ml Sodium heparin, 100 IU/ml Penicillin and 100 µg/ml Streptomycin)

- Cetyl trimethyl ammonium bromide (CTAB) - 0.02%
- TMB/H_2O_2 (Genei, India)
- Sulphuric acid – 2N
- Trypan blue

Procedure

1. 125µl of HBSS (for blank)/CTAB is added to 25µl of cell suspension (2.5×10^7 cells/ml) in 96 well microtitre plate
2. The plate is incubated for 20 min at 30° C

3. To this, 50µl of TMB/H$_2$O$_2$ is added
4. After 2min, 50µl of H$_2$SO$_4$ (2N) is added
5. The plate is centrifuged at 600g for 15 min
6. 200µl of yellow coloured supernatant is transferred to another microtitre plate and OD is read at 450nm.

References

1. Palic, D., Andreasen, C.B., Menzel, B.W. and Roth, J.A. (2005). A rapid, direct assay to measure degranulation of primary granules in neutrophils from kidney of fathead minnow (*Pimephales promelas* Rafinesque, 1820). Fish and Shellfish Immunology 19,217-227.
2. Palic, D., Andreasen, C.B., Menzel, B.W. and Roth, J.A. (2005). A rapid, direct assay parameter in common carp, *Cyprinus carpio*, following herbal treatment for *Aeromonas hydrophila* infection. Aquaculture, 221, 41–50.
3. Alexander CP, Kirubakaran CJ, Michael RD. Water soluble fraction of *Tinospora cordifolia* leaves enhanced the non-specific immune mechanisms and disease resistance in *Oreochromis mossambicus*. Fish Shellfish Immunol. 2010 Nov; 29(5):765-72. doi: 10.1016/j.fsi.2010.07.003.
4. Christybapita D, Divyagnaneswari M, Michael RD. Oral administration of Eclipta alba leaf aqueous extract enhances the non-specific immune responses and disease resistance of Oreochromis mossambicus. Fish Shellfish Immunol. 2007 Oct; 23(4):840-52.
5. Steinhagen D, Helmus T, Maurer S, Michael RD, Leibold W, Scharsack JP, Skouras A, Schuberth HJ. Effect of hexavalent carcinogenic chromium on carp Cyprinus carpio immune cells. Dis Aqua Organ. 2004 Nov 23; 62(1-2):155-61.
6. Prabakaran M, Binuramesh C, Steinhagen D, Michael RD. Immune response and disease resistance of Oreochromis mossambicus to Aeromonas hydrophila after exposure to hexavalent chromium. Dis Aqua Organ. 2006 Mar 2; 68(3):189-96.

.... **Notes/Records** ....

12. FURTHER READINGS

1. Garvey JS, Cremer NE and DH Sussdorf (1977) Methods in Immunology, Third Edition, Benjamin/Cummings Publishing Company, Massachusetts, USA

2. Hudson L and FC Hay (1989) Practical Immunology III edition, Blackwell Scientific Publications, Oxford, London

3. Jolles P. & Jolles J. (1984) What's new in lysozyme research? Always a model system, today as yesterday. Molecular and Cellular Biochemistry pp 63, pp. 165-189.

4. Jolles P. (1969) Lysozymes: a chapter of molecular biology. Angewandte Chemie 8, pp. 227-239.

5. Maxey K.M, Maddipati K.R. and Birkmeier J. (1992). Interference in enzyme immunoassays. Journal of Clinical Immunoassay. 15, 116-120.

6. Myers RL (1989) Immunology a laboratory manual, Wm. C. Brown Publishers Dubuque, Iowa, USA

7. Ossermann E.F. & Lawlor D.P. (1966) Serum and urinary Lysozyme (muramidase) in monocytic and monomyelocytic leukemia. Journal of Experimental Medicine 124, pp. 21-51.

8. Parry R.M., Chandau R.C. & Shahani R.M. (1965) A rapid and sensitive assay of muramidase. Proceedings of the Society for Experimental Biology and Medicine 119, pp.384-386.

9. Salton M.R.J. (1957) The properties of lysozyme and its action on microorganisms. Bacteriological Reviews 21, pp. 82-99.

10. Stolen JS, Fletcher TC, Anderson DP, Roberson BS and WB Van Muiswinkel (1990) Techniques in Fish Immunology FITC-1 SOS publications, Fair Haven, NJ, USA

11. Stolen JS, et al (1992) Techniques in Fish Immunology FITC-2 SOS publications, Fair Haven, NJ, USA

12. Stolen JS, et al (1994) Techniques in Fish Immunology FITC-3 SOS publications, Fair Haven, NJ, USA.

13. APPENDIX

13.1   FISH KEEPING

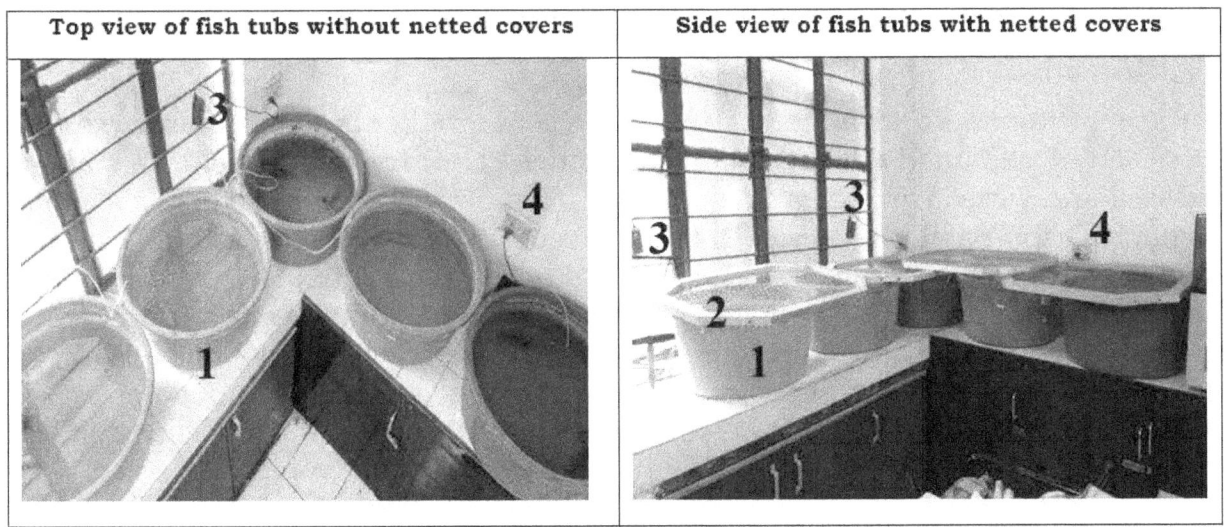

Top view of fish tubs without netted covers	Side view of fish tubs with netted covers

1. Circular plastic tubs (70L), 2. Netted covers for tubs,
3. Aquarium aerators, 4. Electrical point

Requirements

1.   Space – approximately 60 - 80sq.ft with electrical and water connections.
2.   Circular Plastic tubs, volume approximately 70litres, 6- 10nos (Rs. 300 – 500 each). In this tub 5-7 fishes can be maintained.

   Rectangular Fibre Reinforced Plastic (FRP) tanks, 150litres can also be used to keep fish. FRP tanks, 300/500 litres can be used stock fishes (FRP tanks: Trishool agencies, Chennai – Mr. Athi Raman 9176138537)
3.   Fish Tub covers (to be fabricated) made of nylon fish net with large mesh size (fitted in square/octagon frames of PVC or Aluminium, 26" x 26") to prevent fish from jumping out.
4.   Small aerators, minimum 5 numbers to aerate 10 tubs (Rs. 250-400 each).

   Basic maintenance of fish includes daily feeding the fish *ad libitum* with feed (prepared at the lab or purchased) at least once (at the level of 2-4% of body weight per day), daily removing (siphoning out) faecal matter and excess feed from the bottom of fish tanks, alternate day replacing of at least 50% of fish tank water with fresh water and continuous aeration by aerators.

13.2 FISH FEED PREPARATION

Ingredients (for 1 kg of feed)

- Dried fish – 420 g
- Groundnut oil cake – 200 g
- Tapioca flour – 150 g
- Wheat flour – 150 g
- Blood meal – 50 g
- Mineral mix – 20 g
- Vitamins – 10 g

Except vitamins and mineral mix, all other ingredients listed above were dried and powdered separately using a mixer grinder. The dry powdered materials were mixed well and sieved through a fine strainer. This powder [put in an autoclavable bag (HiMedia HiDispo Bag)] was sterilized (using autoclave/pressure cooker for 7 minutes). Then the powder is mixed well with vitamins and mineral mix. Now sterile water is added to this mixture in the ratio of 300 ml of water to 1kg powder and mixed well. Then this 'dough' is pressed through fine pored plate of presser (Ojhas/Anjali to get 'noodles' or 'vermicelli' which is spread on clean sheets paper. Then noodles are dried in shade for a day or two (or at 40 °C for 2-3 hours) till it becomes brittle and stored in airtight box.

Prepared fish feed can be stored for a month at room temperature (for a couple of months if stored at 10 °C (refrigerator). The biochemical analysis of the feed shows protein: 39%; lipid: 11%; water: 10%; ash: 9%and trace amounts of vitamins and minerals.

13.3 FISH PROCURING

Oreochromis mossambicus (Mozambique tilapia) or

Oreochromis niloticus (Nile Tilapia)

Size – 30 – 40 g

Mozambique tilapia is inexpensive and since the fish is invasive, it should be available in any water body, like small or large ponds and lakes in the outskirts of the city. It is poor man's fish and available for a throw away price (Rs.20 or 30 per kg). By contacting a local fish farmer, live fish can be collected and brought in a bucket or polythene bag with water to the laboratory without much problem.

Nile Tilapia can be purchased from willing Nile tilapia farmers at the rate of about Rs.200/kg or Rs. 20 or 30 per fish of 40gm size.

International users of this manual can approach their national or provincial fisheries department for procuring tilapia (tilapia is being cultured throughout the world).

Where to get further information for procuring fish in India and elsewhere?

Contact

Mr. S. Vaitheeswaran

Mr. S. Alagu Ravi

Partners

Svara Biotechnovations

10, Pioneer Avenue,

New Natham Road,

Madurai – 625014, Tamil Nadu, India

Email id: svarabiotechnovations@gmail.com

Mobile No. 09791742398, 09003381453

Phone no: +91 – 452 – 4522398

Centre for Fish Immunology

School of Life Sciences

Vels University

Pallavaram, Chennai-600117 Email id : dinakaranmichael2000@gmail.com

        rdmichael2000@yahoo.co.in

Mobile No. 9842168018, 9962506248

Phone No. +91-44-22662523, 22662500

You may also contact...

Local fish farmers in your district and/or State Fisheries Departments in your District of your State.

13.4   CONSULTANTS FOR IMMUNOTECHNIQUES USING FISH MODEL

Following is the list of Qualified Consultants whom you may consult for any issue in introducing Immunology laboratory exercises using fish model in your curriculum/ programme.

1. **Prof. Dr. R. Dinakaran Michael Ph.D.,**
Dean of Life Sciences and
Director, Centre for Fish Immunology,
Vels Institute of Science, Technology and Advanced Studies,
Pallavaram, Chennai,
Tamil Nadu-600117
Phone: (O) +91-44-22662500, 22662523 (Direct)
(H) +91-44-43863831
Mobile: 98421-68018
Fax: +91-44-22662513
Email: dinakaranmichael2000@gmail.com; rdmichael2000@yahoo.co.in
Website: www.velsuniv.ac.in/centre-fish-immunology.asp

2. **Mr. R. Isaac Arun Kumar, M.Sc.**
Administrator,
The American College Satellite Campus,
Chatrapatti, Madurai,
Tamil Nadu– 625014
Mobile: 09942795690
Email: isaac_arun71@yahoo.com

3. **Dr. Mookkan Prabakaran Ph.D.,**
Principal Investigator,
Molecular viral Pathogenesis,
Temasek Life Sciences Laboratory,
Singapore.
Email: prabha_26@yahoo.com

4. **S/Lt. Dr. C. Binu Ramesh Ph.D.,**
Assistant Professor in Zoology,
PG & Research Department of Zoology and Microbiology,
Thiagarajar College,
Madurai,
Tamil Nadu-625009
Email: binuramesh@gmail.com
        binuramesh@yahoo.com

5. **Dr. L.D. Devasree Ph.D.,**
Assistant Professor, Dept. of Zoology & Head, Dept. of Biotechnology,
The Madura College (Autonomous),
Madurai,
Tamil Nadu-625011
Mobile: 9364215879
E-mail: ganeshkumar.devasree@gmail.com; devamdu@yahoo.co.in

6. **Dr. Catherine P. Alexander Ph.D.,**
Associate Professor,
Research Department of Zoology,
Jayaraj Annapackiam College for Women,
Periyakulam, Theni Dist,
Tamilnadu- 625601
Mobile: 9487582969
E-mail: catherine_ruskin@yahoo.co.in

7. **Dr. M. Divya Gnaneswari Ph.D.,**
Assistant Professor,
Department of Zoology
Gargi College, University of Delhi,
New Delhi – 110049
Email: divyagnaneswari@yahoo.com

8. **Dr. C. JohnWesly Kirubakaran Ph.D.,**
QC – Microbiology, Human Biologicals Institute,
National Dairy Development Board,
The Nilgiris,
Tamil Nadu–-643007
Mobile: 8754574544
E-mail: micjohn@gmail.com

9. **Dr. Priyatharsini Rajendran Ph.D.,**
Associate Professor,
PG Department of Zoology,
Lady Doak College, Madurai,
Tamil Nadu-625002
Mobile no. 9486071644.
Email:priyatharsinirajendran@ldc.edu.in

10. Dr. B. Ramalakshmi M.Sc.,

Centre for Fish Immunology,

Vels Institute of Science, Technology and Advanced Studies,

Pallavaram, Chennai,

Tamil Nadu– 600117

Phone 9488400696

Email b.ramalks@gmail.com

11. Ms. S. Kalaivani Priyadarshini M.Sc., M.Phil.,

Assistant Professor,

Department of Biotechnology,

Lady Doak College,

Madurai,

Tamil Nadu- 625002

Mobile: 9442983746

Email: kalaivanipriyadarshini@ldc.edu.in

12. Mr. A.S. Parasuraman M.Sc.,

DBT-SRF, Ph.D. Scholar,

Centre for Fish Immunology,

Vels Institute of Science, Technology and Advanced Studies,

Pallavaram, Chennai,

Tamil Nadu- 600117

Ph. +91-9840588564.

Email: parasuraman2187@gmail.com

13. Ms. Omita Yengkhom M.Sc.,

Research scholar,

Centre for fish immunology,

Vels Institute of Science, Technology and Advanced Studies,

Pallavaram, Chennai,

Tamil Nadu-600117

Email: omita@velsuniv.org

14. Ms. K.S. Shalini M.Sc.,

Research scholar,

Centre for Fish Immunology,

Vels Institute of Science, Technology and Advanced Studies,

Pallavaram, Chennai,

Tamil Nadu– 600117

Email: shalini86.s@gmail.com

15. Dr. G Raghavendrudu Ph.D.,

Associate Professor,

Dept of Biotechnology,

MITS college of engineering,

Rayagada,

Odisha 765017

Phone 9437908959

Email raghumangrove@gmail.com

16. Dr. Sudhir Verma Ph.D.,

Assistant Professor,

Department of Zoology,

Deen Dayal Upadhyaya College,

(University of Delhi)

Sector-3, Dwarka,

New Delhi-110 078

Phone: 9873566090

Email: sudhirvermazoology@gmail.com; sv_du@yahoo.co.in

17. Dr. Sathya Prasad, N., Ph.D.,

Assistant Professor,

Department of Biochemistry,

Vels Institute of Science, Technology and Advanced Studies,

Pallavaram, Chennai,

Tamil Nadu-600 117

Phone: 07358509785; 09481530132

Email: sathya1prasad@gmail.com

18. Dr. Ivan Aranha Ph.D.,

Zoology Department,

Ahmednagar College,

Ahmednagar,

Maharashtra - 414001

Phone:9766144552/9845700052

Email: ivanaranha@gmail.com

19. Dr. Joe Prasad Mathew Ph.D.,

Associate Professor,

Department of Zoology,

St. Berchmans' College (Autonomous),

Changanacherry, Kottayam (Dist),

Kerala- 686101

Mobile: 9447595916

Email: jopmat@gmail.com

20. Dr. Nageswara Rao Amanchi Ph.D.,

Assistant professor,

Freshwater Ecology @ Aquatic toxicology lab,

Department of zoology,

Nizam College (A), Osmania University,

Basheerbagh, Hyderabad,

Telangana State - 500001

Mobile number@+91-9948902683

Email: bowmibannu@gmail.com; nageswar_ou@yahoo.co.in

21. Dr. M.S.A. Muthukumar Nadar Ph.D.,

Assistant Professor,

Department of Biotechnology,

School of Biotechnology and Health Sciences,

Karunya University,

Coimbatore,

Tamil Nadu-641114

Mobile: +91 9566210873

Email: muthukumar@karunya.edu

22. Ms. M. Indiraleka M.Sc.,

Assistant Professor,

Department of Biotechnology,

Mepco Schlenk Enginerring college,

Sivakasi,

Tamil Nadu– 626005

Mobile no: 7402389414

Email: indira.leka@yahoo.com indirajith1812000@gmail.com

23. Dr. Yumnam Lokeshwor Singh, Ph.D.

Associate Professor,

Department of Zoology,

School of Biological Science,

University of Science & Technology Meghalaya,

Meghalaya – 793101

Contact no: +91 9612253665

Email: lokeyum24@gmail.com

24. Dr. R. Mala Ph.D.,

Associate Professor,

Mepco Schlenk Engineering College,

Sivakasi,

Tamil Nadu– 626005

Email: maalsindia@gmail.com

25. Dr. Nagalakshmi. N. Ph.D.,

Assistant Professor,

Dept. of Microbiology,

Melaka Manipal Medical College (Manipal Campus)

Manipal University, Manipal,

Karnataka

Email: nagubrp@gmail.com

26. Jagnyeswar Ratha, Ph.D.

Lecturer, School of Life Sciences,

Sambalpur University, Jyoti Vihar,

Odisha -768019

Phone: (+91) 94380 60735

Email: jagnyeswar@yahoo.co.in

27. **Mr. G. Arunkumar M.Sc.,**
Department of Biotechnology,
Bannari Amman Institute of Technology,
Sathyamangalam,
Tamilnadu- 63840
Email: arunibt11@gmail.com

28. **Dr. Gayathri Gururajan Ph.D.,**
Assistant Professor,
Department of Microbiology,
School of Life Sciences,
Vels Institute of Science, Technology and Advanced Studies,
Chennai,
Tamil Nadu– 600117
Email: gayathrig.sls@velsuniv.ac.in

29. **Dr. Rajasekaer Thirunavukkarasu Ph.D.,**
Scientist-B,III Floor,
Centre for Drug Discovery and Development,
Col. Dr. Jeppiaar Research Park
Sathyabama University, Jeppiaar Nagar,
Rajiv Gandhi Road,
Chennai,
Tamil Nadu-600 119
Ph: 9751236647 9884826998
Email: microraja09@gmail.com

30. **Dr. Ishtapran Sahoo Ph.D.,**
Assistant Professor,
Department of Biotechnology,
Dayananda Sagar College of Engineering,
Shavige Malleshwara Hills,
Kumarswamy Layout, Bangalore,
Karnataka– 560078
Email: ishtapran@gmail.com

31. **Dr. Narendra Maddu Ph.D.,**
Assistant Professor,
Room No:205, Dept Of Biochemistry,
Sri Krishnadevaraya University,
Anantapur
Karnataka-515003
Email: dr.narendramaddu@gmail.com

32. **Dr. K. Radhakrishnan, Ph.D.,**
Associate Professor and Head,
PG and Research Department of Zoology,
Government Arts College (Autonomous),
Karur,
Tamil Nadu-639005
Ph: 9443882951
Email: ragovila@gmail.com

33. **Dr. G. Bupesh, Ph.D.,**
Senior Research Scientist,
Research & Development Wing,
Sree Balaji Medical College and Hospital,
(A Medical Campus of Bharath University)
No.7 CLC Works Road,
Chromepet, Chennai
Tamil Nadu-600 044
Mobile: 8012405965
Email Id: bupeshgiri55@gmail.com

34. **Dr. B. Meena, Ph.D.,**
Associate professor, Department of Zoology,
Presidency college,
Chennai,
Tamil nadu-600005
Mobile: 7338878098
Email : meena_sk2007@hotmail.com

35. Dr.S.Venkatalakshmi

Associate Professor of Zoology,
Government College for women (A)
Kumbakonam,
Tamil Nadu- 612001
Ph. 09442647313
Email. dr.s.venkatalakshmi@gcwk.ac.in

36. Ms. S. M. Logambal

J-1, Sical Race View Apartment
Race Course Road Interior
Guindy, Chennai,
Tamil Nadu-600032
Mobile:9842956827
E-mail:loge_sm@yahoo.com

13.5 PREPARATION OF REAGENTS

1. **Phosphate Buffered Saline (pH 7.2)**
   - Sodium chloride 8 gm
   - Anhydrous dibasic disodium hydrogen phosphate (Na_2HPO_4) 1.15 gm
   - Anhydrous monobasic potassium dihydrogen phosphate (KH_2PO_4) 0.2 gm
   - Potassium chloride 0.2 gm

   Dissolve above listed chemicals in 900 ml of water with constant stirring. Add distilled water to make it up to 1000 ml and autoclave at 15 pounds for seven minutes.

2. **Alsever's solution**
   - Dextrose 2 g
   - Tri-sodium citrate dehydrate 0.8 g
   - Citric acid monohydrate 0.055 g
   - Sodium chloride 0.42 g
   - Distilled water 100 ml

   The above listed ingredients are dissolved in 100ml of distilled water and the pH is adjusted to 6.1 with 10% citric acid solution and autoclaved at 15 pounds in a pressure cooker for 7 minutes

3. **Hank's balanced salt solution (HBSS without Ca^{++} and Mg^{++}) (pH 7.3)**
   - Sodium chloride 8 g
   - Potassium chloride 0.4 g
   - Anhydrous monobasic potassium phosphate 0.06 g
   - Sodium bicarbonate 0.35 g
   - Anhydrous dibasic sodium phosphate 0.048 g
   - D-glucose 1 g
   - Distilled water 1000 ml

   The above listed ingredients were dissolved in one litre of distilled water and autoclaved at 15 pounds in a pressure cooker for 7 minutes.

4. **Phenol Red Free Hank's balanced salt solution (with Mg^{++} and EGTA)**
   - Sodium chloride 8 g
   - Potassium chloride 0.4 g
   - Anhydrous potassium dihydrogen phosphate (KH_2PO_4) 0.06 g
   - Sodium bicarbonate 0.35 g
   - Anhydrous disodium hydrogen phosphate (Na_2HPO_4) 0.048 g
   - D-glucose 1 g
   - $MgCl_2.6H_2O$ 0.1 g
   - EGTA 10mM

- Distilled water 1000 ml

5. 0.05 M Sodium phosphate buffer (pH 6.2)

Dissolve 6.899 g of Sodium dihydrogen phosphate ($NaH_2PO_4.2H_2O$) in 1000 ml of distilled water. Dissolve 7.098 g Disodium Hydrogen phosphate (Na_2HPO_4) in 1000 ml of distilled water.

Mix 81.5ml of NaH_2PO_4 solution with 18.5ml of Na_2HPO_4 solution and make upto 200ml.

6. Physiological saline

- Sodium chloride 0.87 g
- Distilled water 100 ml

Dissolve Sodium chloride in 90 ml of water with constant stirring. Add enough distilled water to make 100 ml and autoclave at 15 pounds in a pressure cooker for 7 minutes.

7. Carbonate-bicarbonate buffer (pH 9.6)

- Sodium carbonate 1.59 gm
- Sodium bicarbonate 2.93 gm
- Distilled water 1000 ml.

Dissolve the reagents in 900 ml of water with constant stirring. Adjust the pH to 9.6. Add distilled water to make 1000 ml.

8. 0.1 M Succinate Buffer (pH 4.15)

- Succinic acid 11.8 g
- Sodium azide 0.1 g
- Distilled water 1000 ml

9. 1.5% agarose in PBS

- Agarose 1.5g
- Phosphate buffered saline 100ml

The agarose is melted by heating slowly till it dissolves completely and becomes clear.

10. Coomassie staining solution

- 0.1% Coomassie brilliant blue R-250
- 40% Ethanol
- 10% Acetic acid

Dissolve Coomassie brilliant blue R-250 in ethanol before adding acetic acid and water. The solution requires stirring for 1-2 hrs.

www.ingramcontent.com/pod-product-compliance
Lightning Source LLC
Chambersburg PA
CBHW081342180526
45171CB00006B/583